SLEEP - PHYSIOLOGY, FUNCTIONS, DREAMING AND DISORDERS

HENRI PIÉRON AND NATHANIEL KLEITMAN, TWO MAJOR FIGURES OF 20TH CENTURY SLEEP RESEARCH

SLEEP - PHYSIOLOGY, FUNCTIONS, DREAMING AND DISORDERS

Additional books in this series can be found on Nova's website under the Series tab.

Additional e-books in this series can be found on Nova's website under the e-book tab.

SLEEP - PHYSIOLOGY, FUNCTIONS, DREAMING AND DISORDERS

HENRI PIÉRON AND NATHANIEL KLEITMAN, TWO MAJOR FIGURES OF 20TH CENTURY SLEEP RESEARCH

CLAUDE GOTTESMANN

New York

Library of Congress Cataloging-in-Publication Data

Library of Congress Control Number: 2013939133

ISBN: 978-1-62618-990-4

Published by Nova Science Publishers, Inc. † New York

To Cédric, Anne, Julian, Tom

Contents

Abstract

During the twentieth century, only two researchers published world famous, encyclopedic monographs related to sleep. The first of these works appeared in 1913, when Henri Piéron published *"Le problème physiologique du sommeil",* which is still a standard reference today. Although multiple researchers and clinicians, such as Economo (1917, 1928), Berger (1929), Hess (1931), Bremer (1935, 1936), Loomis et al. (1937) and Ranson (1939), subsequently published highly important findings on sleep-waking processes, the next fundamental phase was marked by the publication of the first edition of *Sleep and Wakefulness*, by Nathaniel Kleitman in 1939. Later, following his discovery of the rapid eye movement (REM) dreaming sleep stage in 1953, Kleitman published the masterful second edition of this work in 1963. Later on, several researchers published highly important reviews (Jouvet 1962, 1972, Moruzzi 1963, 1972, Hobson 1988, Steriade and McCarley 1990), although they were directed to more limited topics. Here, we provide an overview of Piéron's and Kleitman's sleep-related papers, placed in their proper historical context.

Keywords: Biological rhythm, BRAC, dreaming, paradoxical sleep, reflexes, REM sleep, Sleep, Sleep deprivation, sleep factor, temperature

Introduction

Nathaniel Kleitman (1895-1999) was one of the major sleep researchers of the last century. In addition to his discovery of the rapid eye movement (REM) dreaming sleep stage in 1953, he is particularly known for the two editions of his famous book "*Sleep and wakefulness*" (Kleitman, 1939, 1963). Following his death in 1999, a commentator stated that "Nathaniel Kleitman is universally recognized as the father of sleep research". (Editorial, 1999). While we do not want to be drawn into an argument on this issue, we would like to point out that the first world-famous sleep researcher and author of the last century was Henri Piéron (1881-1964). Piéron's work, "*Le problème physiologique du sommeil*" (Piéron, 1912), is still sometimes quoted today, although it has been neither translated nor analyzed in details. Published in 1913 (Piéron 1913a), this encyclopedic work analyzed all of his earlier published research on sleep, integrating it into the then-existing knowledge of sleep-waking behavior.

We intend to review the work of Piéron and Kleitman on sleep. Since in *Le problème physiologique du sommeil* and in *Sleep and wakefulness* it is not always easy to dissociate the authors' assertions from those of the broader scientific community, and since in some cases the experimental descriptions given in their respective books lack detail, we decided to analyze all of these authors' successive papers devoted to sleep to follow authors evolution of ideas placed in their proper historical context, beginning with Piéron, who was Kleitman's predecessor. The authors will be quoted directly from their original articles as often as possible.

Henri Piéron

Chapter 1

Henri Piéron

Henri Piéron was born in Paris in 1881. He studied at the Sorbonne and obtained first the "Licence" and then the "Agrégation" (a high-level competitive exam used for teacher recruitment) in Philosophy in 1903, "after a majority (of the examiners), needing to give a score for a lesson of between 2 and 18, settled on a relatively high one to ensure that I would pass" (p 8) (Piéron, 1965). In 1901, at the age of 19, he presented his first communication at the 4th International Congress of Psychology, with the following title: "*Sur l'interprétation des faits de rapidité anormale dans le processus d'évocation des images*" (On the interpretation of abnormal speed in the process of image evocation). (Piéron 1901) (Le Grand 1966) indicating his early interest in visual processes. From the beginning, he fought against the notion that Psychology should be subordinated to Philosophy within academia. As one of the founders of the field of experimental psychology in France (Toulouse, Vaschide and Piéron, 1904), from 1904 onwards he devoted his energies to the promotion of psychology as the objective study of behavior integrated within the biological sciences, but without reducing psychology to physiology (Fessard, 1951). (Figure 1).

Early in his career, Piéron performed research on the lower species in marine laboratories (see below) and, belonging to the Physiological Psychology Laboratory at the Sorbonne (directed by Léon Binet), he worked at the convergence of the laboratory-hospital-natural methods of behavioral studies. "He was convinced that every general law in human psychology is common both to animal and man" (p 149) (Piaget, 1966). He worked with N. Vaschide, under the responsibility of E. Toulouse, later publishing with him and also worked with R. Legendre, essentially on sleep. He defended his thesis in 1912 (Piéron, 1912), the same year he also became a Medical Doctor. After the premature death of Léon Binet in 1911, he became a Professor at the Sorbonne and the director of the Physiological Psychology Laboratory. Continuing Beaunis and Binet's work, he edited the journal "*L'Année Psychologique*". He pursued this work for several decades, during which he wrote numerous analyses and commentaries for the journal.

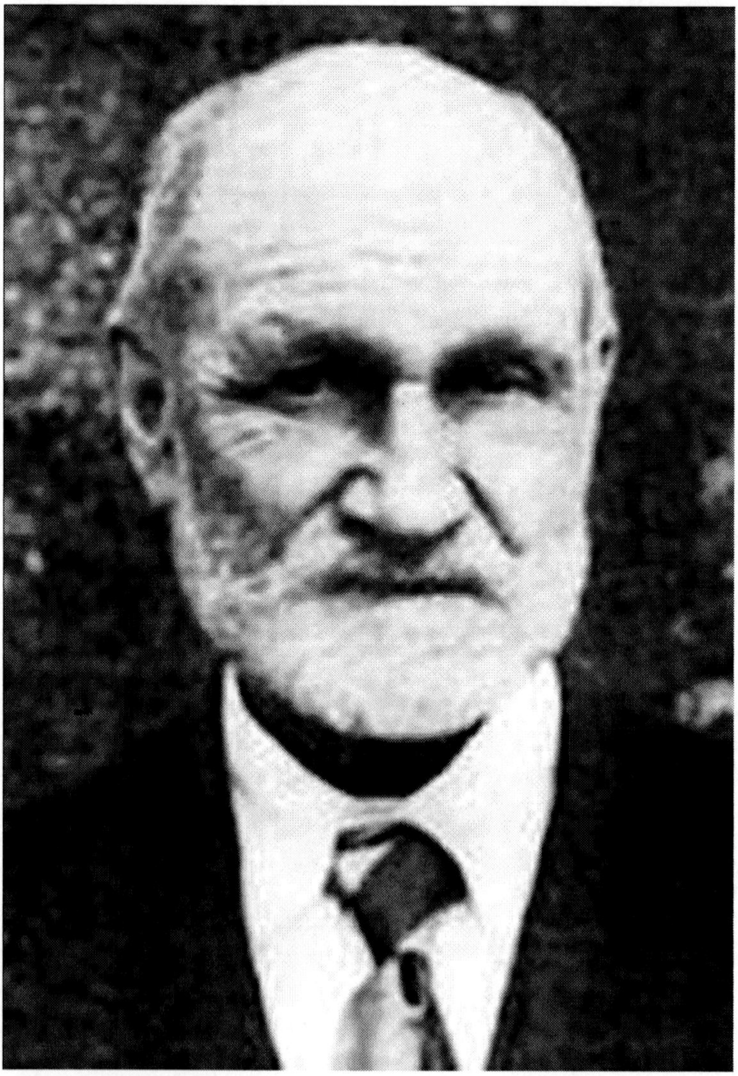

Figure 1. Henri Piéron. Reprinted from *L'Année Psychologique*.

In 1921, he created the first French Institute of Psychology, in Paris, and in 1923 (at the age of 42) he obtained the Chair of Sensory Physiology at the Collège de France; this was to be his primary future field of investigation. The epigraph for his candidature was Johannes Müller's statement "*Nemo psychologus, nisi physiologus*": "One is not a psychologist who is not also a physiologist". In 1928, Piéron was involved in the creation of the National Institute of Professional Orientation, and at the end of WWII, in 1944, he first helped create a certificate in Psychophysiology at the Science Faculty, and then an Arts degree in Psychology that encompassed this certificate. (Reuchlin, 1965).

In a fine and detailed analysis, Georgiade (1970) underlined the pre-cybernetic elements in Piéron's work, such as when he wrote "Psychic processes are essentially processes of nervous influx between fixed elements that constitute (a collection of) posts that can do nothing in isolation" (p 249) (Piéron, 1958). "According to him, the sensory organs, resembling microphones, photoelectric cells, or pH detectors, transform highly varied phenomena into telegraph-like signals… Through his accurate predictions and intuition, Piéron anticipated the development of biocybernetics." (p 174-175) {Georgiade, 1970). Finally, Fraisse (1970) and Littman (1971) discussed the respective roles of Piéron and Watson in the development of the concept of behaviorism. As stated by Littman, "Piéron is to be numbered among those having the honor of very early seeing the methodological significance of behavior-indexing of psychological concepts. However, there is more to history than bestowing honor so we are left with the question of why it is Watson (1913) rather than Piéron, Pavlov (1954) or Bechterew (1913) who is created as the founder of psychological behaviorism" (p 263).

It can only be stated that, as noted above, Henri Piéron founded the field of French scientific psychology in 1904 and thereafter began searching for the physiological basis of behavior. Although Watson is said to have had conversations about behaviorism as early as 1903 (Watson, translation 1972), his first paper was published in 1913, whereas Piéron had defined psychology as the objective study of behavior before then (in at least 1908) (Piéron, 1908e). Among those who early on recognized Piéron as a major international researcher involved in the study of the biological basis of psychology, an anonymous Romanian paper from 1939 must be underlined. We propose as one possible author the editor of the journal in which the paper was published (Stefanescu-Goanga, 1939).

Chapter 2

Piéron's Research on Sleep

Knowledge on Sleep in 1900

Several major papers had been published in the years before Piéron first became involved in his sleep studies. One of them was devoted to sleep deprivation, a main topic of his future research. In that study, Manaceine (1894) had shown that complete sleep deprivation in young dogs induced temperature and blood disturbances, and ultimately death after 92 to 143 hours, confirming a previous observation of human agrypnia (death after 9 days) (Hammonds 1880). A review on this topic had also appeared several years before the end of the century (Patrick and Gilbert 1896). Another significant result was the observation that decorticated dogs showed alternating periods of sleep and wakefulness (Golz 1892). Also, with respect to brain function, it had been shown that brainstem infection at the level of the third nerve nucleus, which was believed to interrupt all sensory afferents, induced sleep: referred to as the "Nona" syndrome (Mauthner 1890), this process was only elucidated much later, following midbrain reticular formation lesions performed in monkeys (Magoun 1948).

Chapter 3

Piéron's Results

In the foreword to his printed thesis, Piéron wrote, on March 6, 1912: "It has now been a dozen years that the question of sleep, in both its physiological and its psychological aspects, has been a subject of preoccupation and of research for me." (p 5) (Piéron, 1913).

Indeed, as early as 1901, at the age of 20, Piéron published two short papers devoted to dreaming; these papers were seemingly performed under the responsibility of N. Vaschide, who contemporaneously published articles on the same topic without Piéron (Vaschide, 1901). At the time, Vaschide was Chef de Travaux and Piéron was demonstrator in the Experimental Psychology Laboratory at the Villejuif Asylum.

The first paper focused on dreaming. "We purpose giving a complete critical exposition of the views which were obtained in Greek and Roman antiquity regarding the prophetic value of dreams" (p 162) (Vaschide and Piéron 1901a). This paper, published in English, was a translation of an unpublished French manuscript. It followed other papers, by Vaschide alone (1899) and by Vaschide and Meunier (1901), which were also devoted to dreaming as well as Ladd's (1892) previous paper. "All dreams are not regarded as having the same standing: there are some which are due to natural influences; the true dreams are those of the morning and of the third watch (Ovid *Metamorph.* XI 633 et seq.) 'because food disturbs dreams' (*Iliad* I, 63)" (p 163) (Vaschide and Piéron 1901a). This beautiful analysis of the ancient literature concluded with assertions like the following: "If we examine the foundations of the belief of the ancients, we shall see that the facts, far from corroborating the belief, owe to the belief whatever validity they possess. In the sequel, they lent some re-enforcement to the belief, but at the origin the belief was far too strong to need their support. For minds who are already absolutely convinced, there is no necessity of proof, and demonstration can come only with criticism… The ancients preferred accepting mistakes made in the interpretation of dreams which were not realized, (and this was the general rule) to renouncing their faith in the prophetic value of dreams, absolutely unfounded though this faith may have been" (p 193) (Vaschide and Piéron 1901a). This highly interesting analysis is Piéron's only English-language paper concerning sleep.

The second paper was a short report on the semiotics of dreams (Vaschide and Piéron, 1901b). It was, to some extent, a continuation of the previous paper. In the report, the authors reported 13 cases in which dreams were premonitory of health disturbances. The method used to collect dream reports was described, and "on average the initial symptoms occurred approximately forty-eight hours after the" dream occurrence (p YY).

In 1902, Vaschide and Piéron published a small book (95 pages) entitled *"La psychologie du rêve au point de vue medical"* ("Dream psychology from a medical perspective"). (Vaschide and Piéron, 1902a). "We view dream psychology from a particular perspective, i.e. semiotics, which is incidentally the only aspect that may be of primary interest to the clinic and to medical science. We therefore do not seek, in these pages, to identify the mechanisms or the intimate structure of normal or pathogenic dreams, and we have left them aside by design (p 5) … The doctor never has too many indices to help in a diagnosis, which is sometimes delicate and difficult; in particular he never has enough precursor symptoms that could allow a precise and early prognosis, especially in certain serious cases. Therefore, we have often spoken of dreams as providers of precious elements, both for diagnosis and for prognosis; and, it is remarkable that we never in fact turn to dreams to obtain such information (p 7) … Their origins … may come from … exterior excitation, a sensation, or even, and it is this final point that interests us, from an internal, organic impression". (p 8). After providing a historical approach to the semiological meaning of dreams, the rest of the book gives numerous examples of dreams followed by: a) general disturbances; b) psychopathologies: "tell me of which you dream, and I'll tell you who you are" (p 43); c) mental alienation; d) hysteria; and e) epilepsy. The authors concluded: "What we would like is to contribute to … finally decide to give, for each disease, alongside the other symptoms, a place for dreams" (p 94)…We would not like to go far beyond the facts that served as premises for the conclusions that we can provide, and yet we do not hesitate to assert that there is truly, in dreams, a precious source, or even a critical source of information, not only regarding our psychological state, but even on our physiological state at the most intimate level, which is expressed in a somehow free way during our sleep, in the subconscious realms of our mind

Nowadays, it is on the unknown realms beneath our consciousness that there is a constant source of contemporary ramblings. Let us say, and let us shine the light of science on these obscure regions to do away with radical superstitions" (p 75). This interest in dreaming, as always (Kant, Schopenhauer, Hughlings Jackson - for reference see Gottesmann 2010), was particularly topical. Indeed, earlier papers had described eye movements and confirmed miosis during sleep (Fontana 1765, Raehlmann and Witkowski 1877, 1878), and had also reported mydriasis during dreaming (Duval 1882). Further, an extensive review on the topic, quoted by Piéron (1912), was published just before the end of the century (Berger and Loewy 1898). Moreover, most likely, as the book was sent for printing in September 1901, the authors were unaware of Freud's psychoanalytic interpretation of dreams (Freud, 1900); the first French translation of Freud's book only appeared in 1926. Three of Freud's papers had already been published in French by the end of the 19th century, possibly explaining Vaschide and Piéron's skepticism toward Freud's theory of unconscious mental processes, even though there is no reference to Freud in their book.

Piéron and Vaschide's second common study concerned observations made on a pair of Siamese twins of Chinese origin (Vaschide and Piéron 1902b). Liao Sienne Chen and Liao Toun Chen were 15-years old and were linked by the abdomen. While this paper primarily addressed the biological and psychological characteristics of the two adolescents, three lines were dedicated to a brief description of their sleep: "The subjects can fall asleep and awake individually; nevertheless, the vast majority of their psychic acts are dictated by a psychological automatism that is admirably and anticipatorily regulated" (p 676) (Vaschide, and Piéron, 1902b). A second (Vaschide and Piéron, 1902c) and third (Vaschide and Piéron, 1902d) paper on the twins were more detailed, focusing on their biological features (blood pressure, respiration, muscular strength, sensory perception and thresholds, behavioral attention, memory) and the relationships between them.

Today, research has shown that although intrinsic electroencephalographic (EEG) characteristics are similar between craniopagus twins during sleep, sleep stage occurrence is independent (Lenard and Schulte 1972, Webb 1978); indeed, in one study the maximum recorded sleep stage correspondence in such twins was only 67% (+/- 5 min) (Lahmeyer 1988).

To conclude this discussion of Piéron's collaboration with Vaschide, interestingly, while Piéron referred to several of their common papers in his thesis, he did not cite their common book on dreaming; also, in the acknowledgments of his thesis, while he thanked Toulouse and Legendre, Piéron did not thank Vaschide (1874-1907). Vaschide died at the age of 33 or 34, although an important book of his appeared several years after his death (Vaschide, 1911) and was republished in 1926. Finally, Nicolae Vaschide, "a meteor in French Psychology" (Michel Huteau), was probably at the origin of Piéron's further interest in the topic of sleep, since he published, without Piéron, several other papers on the psychophysiology of sleep (Vaschide, 1901, Vaschide and Vurpas, 1903).

Piéron's next three papers, all of them co-authored by Toulouse and published in 1906, were related to the inversed temperature rhythms seen in night-time workers. It should be emphasized that, although their research began in 1899, Delczynski (1875) had already described such inversions in humans, and Maurel (1884) had also previously induced the same inversion in animals. Maurel had noted that in animals, "It is readily possible to shift the occurrence of the nyctohemeral (circadian) peak of temperature from the evening to the morning, or vice versa … three competing influences act to bring it about: meals, lighting, and movement. Of these three influences, meals are the most important, to such an extent that even when acting oppositely to the two other factors it still has a dominant effect. The influence of light is manifest, but it only brings about a difference of 0.2°C" (p 588). However, since other authors had been unable to bring about such an inversion, Toulouse and Piéron (1906a) repeated the experiment with nurse volunteers at the mental home in Villejuif. Out of a total of thirteen nurses, seven were included in the experiment. "In the final two, particularly important experiments, lasting respectively for 42 and 64 days, two nurses who had never worked at night were put on the night shift; their temperatures were taken every three hours, and in this way it was possible to follow, day by day, the progressive modifications in their circadian cycles as they adapted to their new way of life" (p 475). In the following issue of the same journal, Toulouse and Piéron (1906b) presented quantitative results from their study (Table 1).

In their third paper, the same authors (Toulouse and Piéron, 1906c) studied the progressive changes in temperature that occur with daytime sleep by the nurses. This example showed the continuous evolution of the nurses from normal night sleep (I) through the successive steps of nighttime work (from II to IV). The total night work period lasted for up to 27 days. The temperature progressively increased at 3:00 and at 6:00 a.m. (Table 2).

Table 1. Body temperature during inversed sleep schedule

Type non inverti.

	Durée moyenne du sommeil.	Températures: 6 h. matin.	Midi.	6 h. soir.	Minuit.
D. (14 jours) . .	5 h. 15	36°53	(Sommeil)	*37°12*	36°66
C. (17 jours) . .	5 h. 45	36°65	(Sommeil)	*37°12*	35°80
Ca. (14 jours). .	5 h. 30	36°85	(Sommeil)	*37°55*	36°81
J. B. (18 jours).	9 heures.	36°86	(Sommeil)	*37°45*	36°86
Moyenne		36°72	»	37°23	36°78

Type inverti.

	Durée moyenne du sommeil.	Températures: 6 h. matin.	Midi.	6 h. soir.	Minuit.
B. (27 jours) . .	6 h. 15	*37°30*	(Sommeil)	36°66	36°62
G. (5 jours). . .	4 heures.	*37°38*	(Sommeil)	36°92	36°65
H. (23 jours) . .	4 h. 30	*37°68*	(Sommeil)	37°12	36°97
Moyenne		37°45	»	36°90	36°75

The non-inversed (top) and inversed (bottom) temperature rhythm in the different nurses at 6.00 a.m., lunch time during sleep, at 6.00 p.m. and at midnight. First column: mean sleep duration. In the nurses with inversed temperature levels, the maximum occurred at 6.00 a.m. and not in the afternoon as usually. Left: subjects and number of days. Moyenne: mean. Reprinted from *Comptes-Rendus des Séances de la Société de Biologie*.

Table 2. Progressive changes in body temperature during inversed sleep schedule

	Température: 6 h. matin.	9 h. matin.	Midi.	3 h. soir.	6 h. soir.	9 h. soir.	Minuit.	3 h. matin.
I. Service de jour (10 jours) . .	*36°61*	36°75	37°03	37°19	37°37	*37°53*	(Sommeil)	
II. 1er service de nuit (1) (8 jours) .	*36°75*	36°80	(Sommeil)		37°24	37°40	*37°53*	36°86
III. 2e service de nuit (9 jours) .	*36°94*	37°04	(Sommeil)		37°21	(37°30)	*37°47*	37°30
IV. 3^e service de nuit (10 jours).	37°04	*36°93*	(Sommeil)		37°12	37°27	37°44	*37°47*

From 6.00 a.m. to 3.00 a.m. the next day. Left: different duration in days for the control (I) and inversed (II to IV) schedules. At 6 a.m. there was a progressive shift from the lowest (36.61°C) to highest (37.04 °C) temperature. Jour: day. Sommeil: sleep. Reprinted from *Comptes-Rendus des Séances de la Société de Biologie*.

When returning to daytime working hours, the recovery of a normal temperature rhythm was also progressive.

In 1907, Toulouse and Piéron published two more papers on the reverse sleep-waking cycle, involving the induction of an inversed circadian temperature rhythm. In the first short report, presented at the Academy of Sciences (Toulouse and Piéron, 1907a), the authors noted that temperatures were measured every six hours and even, in some cases, every three hours. They presented new results concerning periods of inversed sleep that lasted for up to 72 days. As an example, they described three subjects with 55 days of inversion. The temperature of these patients was 37.45°C at 6:00 a.m. and then, following 5 hours of sleep around noon, 36.90°C at 6:00 p.m. and 36.75°C at midnight. In contrast, in non-inverted nurses the temperature was 36.72°C at 6:00 a.m. and 37.23°C at 6:00 p.m. They emphasized that the changes in temperature were progressive and were due to the changes in physical activity. However, since the physical activity involved in nighttime work is less intense than it is during the day shift, and particularly because of the absence of sunlight, the temperature differences observed between the night and the daytime in these subjects were less pronounced than they are during the normal sleep-waking cycle.

The second paper published by Toulouse and Piéron in 1907 was a full-length report (Toulouse and Piéron, 1907b). In it, they added that Delczynski (1875) had studied temperature inversion in bakers, reporting temperatures of 37.8° in the morning and 36.3° in the evening. Referring to Maurel (1884), they also recalled that his inversed temperature results were obtained in rabbits. All of the previously published results to date were detailed. In a discussion of the various factors that are capable of inducing temperature cycle inversion, the authors wrote that it is known that nocturnal birds such as owls have an inversed temperature rhythm, and that while lighting has a thermosthenic function, it is not an important factor, in contrast to physical and mental activity. Finally, the organism adapts only gradually to the inverse activity rhythm, and the modification of the temperature rhythm that follows the adaptation of the central nervous system is slow to stabilize and can only slowly revert to a normal circadian cycle.

In 1907, Piéron also began a major collaboration with Legendre on sleep factors. As there were numerous other papers published in that year, including some by Piéron alone, they are presented chronologically here.

Piéron (1907a) first wrote a commentary on anticipatory physiological phenomena, which are indicators of adaptive processes. This followed up on one of his research projects performed on anemones, as well as on those performed with Toulouse on adaptive temperature processes (see above). Just as anemones close and draw in their tentacles even before ebb tide begins, "we sleep before needing to sleep, and it's this same "luxury" sleep, which is similar to our "luxury" breathing…and "luxury" eating, which was able to justify the success of the interesting theory of sleep presented by Mr. Claparède (1905), a theory whose value lies in the phenomenon of anticipation, acting before the profound causes that justify the need for sleep, under penalty of death (p 87) … "This rhythmicity based on anticipation is a phenomenon that could be called a memory phenomenon, consisting as it does of an adaptive use of the past to determine the future. And therein lies a property that could belong to the nervous system, whether it is diffuse as in protozoans or more or less differentiated as in metazoans." (p 87). However, after a study carried out by other researchers on hepatic cells showing strongly analogous memory phenomena, it could be "a fundamental biological property belonging to all protoplasm." (p 88) (Piéron 1907a).

Also in 1907, Piéron (1907b) wrote a paper on the methodology that he had decided to use for his sleep studies. "I have provisionally left aside the question of the *mechanism* of sleep, focusing exclusively on its *causes*; before seeking to understand how the factors act, it seemed to me useful to first determine what the factors are" (p 308).

> "… At first it might seem tempting to try to determine, following the suggestions of what are by now numerous observations, under what circumstances it is possible to experimentally produce a sleep state and to thus carry out a precise analysis. This path has been tried relatively often, but it has led absolutely nowhere…With anemia or cerebral compression, with various forms of intoxication, with certain cerebral tumors, with trypanosomiasis…under the influence of cold in the mountains ... or of various hypnotics or anesthetics, there appears a state called sleep, which the individual cannot in general avoid…It is possible that the mechanisms used by these diverse factors offer real analogies in their inhibitory actions on the function of certain centers. But nothing allows us to conclude from this anything about the factors that provoke periodic sleep …
>
> … A second method consists then of studying a sleeping animal, to search for the deep modifications that it displays compared to an awake animal, and to analyze these modifications. It is this method that the histologists have turned to, believing that they have observed a retraction of neurons during sleep … In reality, in sacrificed, sleeping animals, there is no modification of cortical cells relative to the cells of an awake animal." Piéron then refers to the work of Stefanowska (1900). … "It thus

becomes necessary, henceforth, to study not daily sleep, which can be avoided, but to study an imperative sleep …

… I was seeking at first to produce an imperative need for sleep by muscular fatigue, by making dogs work on the running wheel. But such fatigue sometimes causes excitation phenomena and does not necessarily lead to a need for sleep (blood from fatigued animals does not reproduce, by injection, symptoms of fatigue in another animal).

… There was only one approach left, consisting of waiting for the imperative need for sleep, by preventing dogs from sleeping without making them physically tired, which I accomplished by entrusting the dogs during the night to the general watchman of the Villejuif asylum, who took the dogs with him as he made his rounds and who did not let them rest, and by attaching them during the day by a chain that was too short to allow them to recline, and by repeated stimulation by a certain number of people, preventing them from becoming sleepy.

… This is the study approach that I adopted. I will present at a future date the series of experiments that I have undertaken and the current state of the question, whose solution I intend to continue pursuing." (p 308-309) (Piéron 1907b). It is of interest that, in fact, Piéron set out to verify a theory that had previously been developed by earlier researchers, postulating that endogenous narcotic compounds in the brain were responsible for sleep similarly to chloroform and morphine: "The narcotic sleep substances first act on the entire nervous system, causing, after a short period of irritation, a decrease in its function, and then interrupt the contiguity of neurons, enhancing this decrease in function." (p 417) (Berger and Loewy 1898).

Piéron, working together with Legendre (Legendre and Piéron 1907a), observed disturbances in primarily cortical pyramidal neurons following experimentally induced sleep deprivation in adult dogs: "Prevented from sleeping from the morning of November 18 until the morning of November 24, 1906, required to walk all night long, attached during the day with a leash too short to permit them from lying down, and kept awake by frequent stimulation by several people." (p 312). The results revealed "a slight increase in the volume of cells and nuclei; decentered nucleoles encompassing multiple non-stainable vacuoles; perinuclear chromatolysis, dendrite varicosities with a vacuolar aspect" (p 312). The dogs displayed a rapid recovery of normal behavior that was already evident after three hours of sleep: "The rapidity of the recovery is remarkable, it can already be detected. Patrick and Gilbert (1896) observed that, after a voluntary insomnia lasting 90 hours, in three men at the limits of their ability to resist, a complete recovery was obtained after sleeping barely four hours beyond their normal daily sleep duration." (p 313).

Legendre and Piéron noted that their neuron results confirmed those of Manaceine (1894) (see also Kovalzon 2012), which were performed on young dogs and which also showed brain cell disturbances.

In the same issue of the same journal, Piéron (1907c) described the method that he was using to study the sleep factors. He noted that, with increased insomnia, there is a progressive increase in the pressure to sleep. For the first time, he wrote about the synthesis of 'hypnotoxins' "whose nature we cannot presume to anticipate in any way" (p 342). "These hypnotoxins must be found either in the general circulation or at their site of action, depending on whether they act as exotoxins or endotoxins ... The substances sampled include the blood (either simply defibrinated or also centrifuged, in which case only the serum was used) and the cerebrospinal fluid; the mode of administration was either intravenous, arterial, spinal, ventricular, or cerebral ... The operations were performed, naturally, without general anesthesia, but with a cocaine-based local anesthetic ... Fluid from sleep-deprived dogs was never introduced multiple times into the same dog, in order to avoid potential immunization against hypothetical hypnotoxins. Finally, I relied especially on very young animals, because they proved to be particularly sensitive to the need for sleep ... Experiments carried out following these general guidelines are underway." (p 343-344) (Piéron 1907c). Anticipating later-published results, he already noted the difficulty of the research and the likelihood that the existence of the 'hypnotoxins' would not be ultimately confirmed.

Next, Piéron published two papers devoted to attempts to transfer the sleep-inducing factors. In the first paper Piéron (1907d), he described the difficulties he was encountering. The ventricular route of serum injection (1 cc) did not produce any results, because of drowsiness effects due to compression, with a mechanical effect analogous to several tumors. Injection into the cerebral fluid at the level of the fourth lumbar vertebra space can be done without anesthesia, but did not produce any clear-cut results and was "condemned to ineffectiveness" (p 401). Finally, the intraperitoneal route had no effects in one control animal. Piéron stated that absorption was too slow with this method.

In the second paper, Piéron (1907e) was similarly unable to induce sleep by transferring defibinated blood to the femoral artery. "In all of these experiments, I was unable to provide any evidence in the defibrinated blood of sleep-deprived animals of a hypnotoxic substance capable of reproducing the need for sleep which is so evident in certain cases in sleep-deprived animals ... In experiments that I will describe at a later time, I also carried out intracerebral injections permitting the detection, at minimal doses, of the influence of this particular neurotoxin which would represent, if it exists, the sleep toxin." (p 1006). Thus, in 1907, Piéron generally encountered failure in his hypnotoxin transfer project.

Piéron's subsequent research, performed together with Legendre (Legendre and Piéron, 1907b), compared the pyramidal neurons of the frontal cortex after sleep deprivation and after sleep recovery. A male dog named Fox was allowed to recover, whereas Finette, a female, was sacrificed after the deprivation. Finette's neurons showed: "reduced cell volume. Shriveled nuclei, often off-center. Dendritic varicosities, intraprotoplasmic vacuoles. Nucleoli often ectopic. Reasonably often, two equal or unequal nucleoli situated at different positions throughout the nucleus. Perinuclear or complete chromatolysis. Numerous glial cells, often with two nucleoli. The cellular modifications most often occur in zones or discrete areas; there are groups of cells that are strongly chromatolytic, or achromatolytic, with others remaining significantly less altered." (p 1008). In contrast, in Fox, after 3 days of recovery, "The exam did not reveal, in those regions showing alterations in Finette, any appreciable modifications" (p 1008).

Finally, the same year, Piéron (1907f) published a commentary on the adaptive biological processes occurring in different species. With respect to survival, he distinguished between reflexive modifications of biological properties by anticipation, such as changes in the color of sole as a function of the sea floor, and periodic rhythmic changes, such as temperature modifications, which take time to adapt to new activity-rest situations and which ultimately return to the normal rhythm when the sleep-waking cycle returns to the original conditions. He wrote about an organic chronometer which would anticipate the disturbance: falling asleep precedes the true need for sleep, and respiration occurs prior to the accumulation of CO_2. "There is, in these anticipatory adaptation phenomena, the use of the past to determine the future in a way that is advantageous for the organism, and it is used fully at all levels of differentiation and of evolution, from the nerve cell of the anemone (which closes even before the tide falls (Piéron, 1906, Bohn and Piéron 1906) to the cerebral centers of man, from a reaction to the tides to our own scientific foresight" (p 340) (Piéron 1907f). Thus, these general adaptive processes involve memory phenomena and some degree of inertia.

In 1908, Piéron (1908a) published a short commentary on the polygenesis of sleep states. He defined sleep as states "where the voluntary relations of an individual with his or her environment (by the phenomena of sensitivity and movement) are more or less completely suspended and which can be divided into states of accidental and periodic sleep" (p 252). There are numerous examples of accidental sleep, resulting from intoxication, exhaustion, cold, air rarefaction, brain tumors, anemia, etc.; these can have various physiological consequences, inducing, for example, cellular asphyxia in anemia and alterations of protoplasm with intoxication. Periodic sleep can be categorized as either seasonal or daily sleep. Seasonal sleep, e.g. winter or summer sleep, can be induced by dryness, absence of food, etc. The influence of these factors is indirect and results from an adaptation of the organism to these conditions through anticipated reactions.

"Finally, there is a truly polygenic sleep, which is an extremely general phenomenon in the zoological world. Indeed, there is a voluntary sleep, a boredom-induced sleep, etc. … which results from a true adaptation of the organism; still, here as well, there is an anticipation to a noxious factor which is the direct inducer of sleep, because experimentally-induced sleep deprivation leads to an imperative need for sleep that ultimately results in coma and death: one is obliged to sleep under penalty of death. This direct factor is not known; it could be a chemical agent (note: this was hypothesized for the first time by Piéron) or the result of an excessive disassimilation occurring during nerve cell function, a disassimilation that causes a need for rest during which the equilibrium of the organic state can be reversed, with the assimilation overcoming the expenditure, and for (the nerve cells') reserves to be reconstituted" (p 253) (Piéron 1908a).

In 1908, Legendre and Piéron (1908) published a paper dealing with the neuron disturbances that can occur with sleep deprivation. While their previous study (Legendre and Piéron, 1907g) had only examined the frontal cortex, in this paper they also presented results involving other brain structures.

A female dog was sleep deprived from March 1 until March 10, when it was sacrificed.

> "The spinal ganglion, examined using Nissl's method, show absolutely normal cells, with centrally located nuclei containing one nucleolus; duplicated nucleoli, or exocentric nucleoli or nuclei, are very rare; the chromatophilic substance is normal, the particles are abundant and well distributed, there are no intracytoplasmic vacuoles …
>
> … The horn cells of the spinal cord and the bulb nuclei are also perfectly normal; none of them presents the slightest abnormality. In the cerebellum, a few Purkinje cells show a slight chromatolysis…
>
> ... As far as the occipital lobe is concerned, normality still appears to be the rule; there is no chromatolysis of cells, the nuclei are centrally

located, the nucleoli are only very rarely exocentric, the glial cells are normal …

… In the region of the gyrus sigmoid, there are relatively clear alterations: the cellular volume is often reduced; the nuclei are occasionally exocentric, as are the nucleoli, although such cases are rare; a few small intraprotoplasmic vacuoles appear in certain cells and, somewhat rarely, dendritic varicosities can be perceived. In the affected cells, what is most evident is the chromatolysis, which is frequent. Around such cells, glial cells are abundant …

… The prefrontal region contains lesions that are much more frequent and much more intense. The cellular volume is very often reduced, the cells appear shriveled, the nuclei and nucleoli are very often exocentric, to the point where the nucleolus sometimes appears to touch the edge of the cell, and appear alone and well defined in sections stained by the Nissl method, due to the sometimes complete achromatosis of the cell body. Chromatolysis is indeed extremely widespread and very intense …

… While dendritic varicosities are relatively rare, the vacuolization of the protoplasma is in contrast very frequent; numerous vacuoles of often considerable volume are visible within the most affected cells, which are surrounded by a multiplicity of glial cells …

… Concerning the cortical distribution, we can note that the most affected cells are invariably the large pyramidal cells; the horizontal cells appear to be hardly affected; the small pyramidal and the polymorphic cells are little altered. Among the large pyramidal cells, there are, in addition, scattered here and there, isolated normal cells located next to the others." (p 1103-1104) (Legendre and Piéron 1908).

This was Piéron's first full description of his histological brain analyses related to sleep deprivation. In the discussion, he mentions the results of two previous studies. In the first, Pugnat (1901) found nearly no disturbances in the pyramidal cells (in contrast to the cells of the superficial layers, which showed chromatolysis and excentric nuclei) in dogs following active sleep deprivation (they were forced to walk from 64 to 93 kilometers on a moving wheel). Second, Piéron mentions Guerrini (1900), who found disturbances in motor cortex cells after sleep deprivation. In the Introduction of their paper, Legendre and Piéron recalled that their previous paper had shown that the disturbances are reversed by sleep recovery.

Again in 1908, Piéron (1908b) performed research on sensitivity in fish and triton. One paragraph was devoted to the sleep of the latter. "During the day, the tritons occasionally come to the surface to breathe (every four minutes on average, between two and eight minutes), making a few lazy swimming movements when they are at the bottom of the aquarium, relatively far from the surface. In the evening, in the dark, or even under a constant source of artificial light, they remain in the upper part of the water, or climb by sticking to the walls of the aquarium, often leaving the water completely; they sleep in this way, with their eyes closed, are difficult to awaken, and at times remain asleep until significantly after daybreak (from 7:00 to 8:00 p.m. until 6:00 to 7:00 a.m." (p 327) (Piéron 1908b).

Finally, in 1908, Piéron (1908c), with his bright intellectual outlook, wrote a powerful review on a totally different topic from sleep regulation. The paper, entitled "*L'évolution du psychisme*", contained ideas and concepts that were advanced for the time, pointing the way to the future field of neuropsychology.

In 1910, Piéron published several papers and a book. The latter, entitled *"L'évolution de la mémoire"* (Piéron, 1910a), was a powerful study that encompassed all of the then-available results related to memory processes. He not only described his own results, but also included a beautiful discussion of the evolution and adaptability of memory processes, from invertebrates up to humans. "Human psychology should benefit from research carried out in animals, just as animal psychology will benefit from research carried out in man." (p 5). Moreover, he insisted on the importance of adaptability linked to the environment. "The modifications that constitute individual acquisitions represent effective adaptations, responding to the experience of animals that learn and perfect their conduct" (p 346). Finally, he concluded with a sentence that is important for modern society: "The excessive strength of social memory becomes truly dangerous for the individual that it imprisons and castrates." (p 351) (Piéron, 1910a).

Again in 1910, Legendre and Piéron (1910a) carried out a study to test the osmotic theory of sleep.

> "Among the uncountable theories of sleep, which naturally honor the rich imagination of their inventors, the most recent tend to explain the facts by a physical action of particular humors in the blood, and in the lymph in particular, on cerebral cells.
>
> These theories seems to have three principal forms:
>
> 1° Sleep is caused by an increase in the viscosity of the blood, which would thus circulate more slowly, rendering cerebral function more difficult.
>
> 2° There is a hypertonia of the blood and the lymph, which become progressively loaded with the byproducts of organismal activity, and this hypertonia interferes with the

function of the cerebral cells and causes the lesions that we have observed in association with an imperative need for sleep.

3° Finally, the hypertonia of the blood could attract water from tissues and in particular dehydrate cerebral cells; sleep would thus be the consequence of cerebral anhydrobiosis.

Since, in the field of biology, it is dangerous to resort exclusively to reasoning, and despite the small likelihood of these explanations, it seemed useful to carry out research in this area.

We used the general method previously presented by one of us, consisting of examining dogs with an extremely intense need for sleep after having been prevented from sleeping day and night for ten days, without muscular fatigue". (p 962) (Table 3).

Table 3. Blood properties after sleep deprivation

Artémis, Setter ♀ 22 kilogrammes (10 jours d'insomnie).

	AVANT	APRÈS	DIFFÉRENCE
Point cryoscopique	— 0°59	— 0°58	— 0°01
Densité	1,064	1,057	— 0,007
Extrait sec – Sang total	?	20,55 p. 100	?
Extrait sec – Sang défibriné	21,4 p. 100	19,25 p. 100	— 2,15 p. 100
Viscosité	2,71	2,0	— 0,71
Quantité de sérum	38 p. 100	45 p. 100	+ 7 p. 100

Douillet, ♂, 26 kilogrammes (10 jours d'insomnie).

	AVANT	APRÈS	DIFFÉRENCE
Densité	1,067	1,059	— 0,008
Extrait sec – Sang total	23,4 p. 100	22,3 p. 100	— 1,1 p. 100
Extrait sec – Sang défibriné	23,2 p. 100	21,5 p. 100	— 1,7 p. 100
Viscosité	2,69	2,46	— 0,43

Results after 10 days sleep deprivation in two dogs. Extrait sec: dry extract. Sang total: total blood. Sang défibriné: defibrinated blood. Avant: before, après: after sleep deprivation. Reprinted from *Comptes-Rendus des Séances de la Société de Biologie*.

The authors next quantified the amount of water contained within the cortical white and grey matter. "There is proportionally less water in the control dog, both in the blood and in the brain, which does not help to confirm the hypothesis of an antagonism in their respective contents. ... In their diverse forms, the so-called osmotic theories of sleep are thus clearly refuted by the experimental data" (p 964) (Legendre and Piéron 1910a).

In 1910, Piéron (1910b) wrote a long paper on the behavior of two mollusks, in which protective immobility, but not resting immobility, is described. In his paper, Piéron refers to other papers, the list of which we provide here, in part to show the breadth of Piéron's interests and knowledge (Bohn and Piéron 1906, Piéron, 1904a,b; 1906, 1907g; 1908e,f,g,h,i; 1909a,b ; 1910c,d,e).

The same year, Legendre and Piéron (1910b) published their first paper on the possibility of inducing sleep through autonarcosis as provoked by carbonic gas (CO_2). The authors quantified the levels of CO_2 and O_2 in the expired air before and after sleep deprivation (Table 4).

Table 4. Expired gas during sleep deprivation in a dog

Artémis. ♀ 22 kilogrammes.

	Air expiré — CO^2	Air expiré — O	Quotient respiratoire.	Nombre de respirations à la minute.
3 novembre 1909, 10 h. mat.	2,9 p. 100	17,0 —	0,74	19
20 novembre 1909, 10 h. mat.	1,5 p. 100	18,1 —	0,53	22
Le sommeil de l'animal est rendu impossible à partir du 20 au soir.				
22 novembre 1909, 9 h. 30 mat.	1,4 p. 100	17,5 —	0,41	18
24 novembre 1909, 5 h. soir	1,5 p. 100	18,0 —	0,51	12
25 novembre 1909, 9 h. 30 mat.	1,4 p. 100	17,6 —	0,42	16
27 novembre 1909. 9 h. 30 mat.	2,1 p. 100	17,2 —	0,56	14
29 novembre 1909, 10 h. mat.	3,0 p. 100	14,8 —	0,49	13
30 novembre 1909, 9 h. 30 mat.	1,5 p. 100	17,7 —	0,47	13

Expired carbonic gas and oxygen prior to and after progressive sleep deprivation. Note the progressive decrease in breathing frequency during deprivation and the nearly unchanged expired gas content during increased sleep deprivation, beginning on November 20. Mat: morning. Soir: evening. Reprinted from *Comptes-Rendus des Séances de la Société de Biologie*.

Similar results were obtained on a second dog.

"There are thus no systematic variations in respiratory exchange during the building up of the need for sleep, which soon becomes irresistible" (p 1015).

The authors also tried to quantify the level of CO_2 in the blood before and after deprivation, in one case finding slightly less CO_2 after deprivation.

> "We are therefore able to confirm that the need for sleep, or more generally normal sleep, is not due to carbonic autonarcosis" (p 1015) (Legendre and Piéron 1910b).

The same year, Legendre and Piéron (1910c) replicated the transfer of blood and brain extracts from sleep-deprived dogs to normal recipients. From 60 to 200 cc of serum were injected into the saphenae of dogs, and control serum from non-deprived dogs was injected into non-deprived animals. With respect to both their sleep-related and their histological results, the authors wrote that "the vascular injections give results that are difficult to interpret" (p 1078).

Next, the authors transferred brain emulsions from sleep-deprived dogs into the frontal brain of normal recipients, performing at the same time a control experiment involving the transfer of emulsion from a non-deprived dog into a normal recipient, with both taking place after trephination. This experiment also failed to give any clear results. "

> "Concerning the intra-cerebral injections, which is a brutal and scarcely physiological approach, it is immediately evident that the experiment can have no meaningful result: its toxic effects appear to diffuse very little and to become localized at the site of injection, and its physiological effects (photophobia and somnolence?) seem to be due to compression phenomena ... In sum, it is impossible to conclude based on these experiments that there is a hypnotoxic influence accompanying the imperative need for sleep in sleep-deprived animals" (p 1079) (Legendre and Piéron 1910c).

In a short communication published the same year, Legendre and Piéron (1910d) also described the subarachnoid transfer of extracts prepared from the homogenized cerebral hemispheres of a sleep-deprived dog ('Artemis'). The brain extracts were injected into 'Jaunet', CSF was injected into 'Blanchard', and serum was injected into 'Agitée'. All injections were performed at 37°C, following the removal of an equivalent volume of ventricular fluid. Extremely pronounced sleepiness was observed in all three animals. The histological analysis revealed the presence of typical frontal lesions, with particularly frequent disturbances among the large pyramidal cells, which showed exocentric nuclei and nucleoli. The temporal and occipital cortices showed almost no disturbances, and the cerebellum appeared entirely unaffected. This was the first positive result showing the successful transfer of a 'hypnotoxic' factor.

Next, cerebral fluid was injected under various conditions: 1/ under the same conditions as in the previous experiments (to 'Follet'); 2/ after incubation at 55° for 3 minutes (to 'Résigné'); 3/ after incubation at 65° for 5 minutes (to 'Trapu'); and 4/ after dialysis (to 'Négrillot'). While strong sleepiness was observed in Follet, this effect was significantly decreased and delayed in Résigné; this decrease in sleepiness was even more pronounced in Trapu and the effect was absent in Négrillot. The histological study revealed clear-cut but low intensity lesions in the frontal cortex of Follet; these were still less pronounced in Résigné (a few large pyramidal cells were disturbed), and no disturbances were observed in Trapu or Négrillot. In the temporal and occipital cortices, there were no disturbances in Follet or Résigné (except in rare large pyramidal cells), and the same was observed in Négrillot. In contrast, in Trapu the large pyramidal cells were very disturbed.

The authors performed three control experiments and observed only slight sleepiness or photophobia. There were no histological lesions.

Finally, a histological analysis was performed on the sleep-deprived animals from the first experiment. There was a clear correlation between the length of the sleep deprivation and the extent of the cell disturbances.

Carefully, the authors called for the replication of these experiments, so that "the question of the imperative sleep factors can enter a new period in which we will no longer need to resort to gratuitous hypotheses" (p 1109) (Legendre and Piéron 1910d).

Accordingly, the next year, Legendre and Piéron (1911a) replicated the experiment. They first took blood and CSF from 'Saint Germain', which had been sleep deprived for 11 days. Then, CSF was removed from 'Crépu', and serum from 'Saint Germain' was injected (at 37°C) at the same location. This induced sleepiness and frontal cortex neuron disturbances (chromatolysis of large pyramidal and polymorph cells). The same procedure was performed in 'Tacheté', although this time using CSF from 'Saint Germain'. This treatment induced exactly the same behavioral and histological effects. Control experiments using normal serum or CSF induced no effects in 'Néra' or 'Remuante', respectively. After heating 'Saint Germain's' serum and CSF to 65°C, there were no effects in 'Griffarde' or 'Poilu', respectively. Finally, normal serum, after heating to 65°C, had no effect on 'Pius'.

> "The imperative need for sleep, which appears during the course of experimentally imposed insomnia, is correlated with the development, in the humors, of hypnotoxic properties having the two-fold effect of provoking in a normal animal an intense need for sleep, with an accompanying loss of sensorial attention and of reactive capacity as well as of motor attention and muscular tonus, and of causing cellular alterations characterized especially by chromatolysis, cellular deformations, and displacement of the nucleus and the nucleoli almost exclusively observed in the large pyramidal and polymorphic cells of the frontal lobe, the specificity of this toxic activity having never been refuted …
>
> … The hypnotoxic activity, which appears to be more intense in the cerebrospinal fluid than in the serum, and which is also found in the cerebral plasma, may be related to the waste products of metabolism of nervous cells in the superior centers" (p 191-192) (Legendre and Piéron 1911 a).

Again in 1911, Legendre and Piéron (1911b) presented a paper at the French Academy of Sciences. They noted that their report encompassed results from six years of research, performed on more than sixty dogs that had been sleep deprived for 8 to 10 days, with the animals never having been muscularly fatigued. They briefly described all of their behavioral and physiological observations: respiration, blood, carbonic acid content of the blood, and water content of the cerebral white matter, all of which were unchanged following sleep deprivation. The authors described the behavioral features of sleepiness that accompanied sleep deprivation, particularly the difficulty in maintaining the waking state. They then described how the transfer of serum, cerebral plasma, or, most significantly, CSF, from sleep-deprived animals into the fourth ventricle (icv) of normal dogs induced sleepiness. Only the large pyramidal and polymorph cells of the frontal cortex were obviously disturbed by the transfer of the sleep factor, which was destroyed at 65°C and which disappeared after dialysis.

It should be added that, in 1911, Legendre (1911) published a long article on sleep by himself. All of the behavioral and physiological data known at the time were taken into account. Among them, he mentioned those obtained with "my friend Piéron" (p 749).

In the same year, Legendre and Piéron (1911c) wanted to definitively verify that sleep deprivation was solely responsible for the histological disturbances observed in their research. They therefore studied the effects of long-duration muscular activity. The authors first noted that they had always studied the behavioral and histological consequences of sleep deprivation, being attentive to avoid any physical tiredness in their dogs. Then, they detailed the results available in the literature, describing how several authors had studied muscular tiredness in different species and had shown, in particular, that in mammals there were no lesions of the frontal cortex neurons. Legendre and Piéron's study was performed on a dog running in a wheel, on brown rats (*Mus decumanus,* now referred to as *Rattus norvegicus*), and on a stag after being hunted by dogs. After the dog had run 50 km, the spinal nodes, the spinal cord (including the motor ventral horn), and the cerebellum were all normal. Three cortical regions were examined: first, the frontal lobe and motor cortex, and then the parietal and occipital lobes. The overall aspects of all three regions were normal; only occasional small and medium-sized pyramidal cells had slightly reduced volumes, exocentric nucleoli, or weak perinuclear chromatolysis. "But these minimal alterations can be observed in normal animals" (p 524). The brown rats were forced to run on a wheel or were agitated in a glass enclosure. On the wheel, the animals ran from 10:00 a.m. until 6:30 p.m. Their spinal cords, medulla oblongata, and brains were all normal. Only the Purkinje cells sometimes showed chromatolysis and exocentric nucleoli. One animal showed motor cortex disturbances, particularly in the deeper layers, while all the other parts of the central nervous system were normal. Two brown rats were agitated in the enclosure for more than 10 hours. No abnormalities were found in their central nervous systems. The stag, examined just after death, showed no disturbances in the brain, medulla oblongata, or spinal cord. "We can satisfactorily conclude, therefore, that physiological muscular fatigue does not produce intense and well defined modifications in the central nervous cells, in contrast to electrical excitation and to strychnine" (which had previously been observed by other researchers) (p 526) (Legendre and Piéron 1911c).

In 1912, Legendre and Piéron (1912a) continued in their attempts to characterize the properties of the so-called hypnotoxin. Three dogs, named 'Robuste', 'Castor' and 'Tunis', were sleep deprived for long periods and showed the now classical symptoms: sleepiness and a strong need for sleep, and afterwards disturbances in the frontal cortex neurons, whereas those of the cross (motor) and occipital cortices were normal. One exception was 'Robuste', which showed no clear-cut tendency to sleep even after 293 hours of sleep deprivation (!) (probably the deprivation had not been complete, see later Kleitman 1927). Then, 'Negrito', a control dog, received serum (at 38°C) from 'Robuste' in the 4th ventricle (icv). The serum induced some sleepiness and some need for sleep; there were no histological disturbances. Another dog, 'Piaillard' received serum at 38°C from 'Castor' (269 h deprivation) and showed sleepiness and a clear-cut need for sleep. Cross and occipital neurons were normal, but there were some perturbations in the frontal cells. Finally, 'Carthage' received serum at 39°C from 'Tunis' (269 h deprivation). In this case, there was a strong need for sleep. Once again, the cross and occipital neurons were intact, whereas the frontal cortex neurons showed strong disturbances. In all cases, an equivalent volume of ventricular fluid was removed from the recipients prior to the injections.

Next, the authors injected CSF into normal dogs. 'Negro' received CSF at 39°C from 'Robuste'. This treatment induced only light sleepiness, without any histological disturbances. 'Teigneuse' received CSF at 39°C from 'Tunis' and showed deep sleepiness. The frontal and occipital neurons were normal, whereas the pyramidal cells of the cortical cross level were disturbed.

The authors next studied the influence of heating. Heating to 55°C for 10 minutes had no effect on the ability of serum obtained from 'Robuste' to induce sleepiness in control 'Maroc' but did not induce neuronal disturbances in the frontal cortex. The same result for sleep was observed, under the same conditions, in 'Vive' after injection of serum from 'Castor', while there were frontal neuron disturbances. In contrast, when CSF from 'Tunis' was maintained at 65°C for 10 minutes, it did not induce sleep in 'Tripoli'.

In addition, CSF from 'Tunis' did not induce any sleepiness in 'Lilli' following ultrafiltration.

They thus concluded,

> "Heating serum to 55 degrees had no effect, while heating to 65 degrees made the hypnotoxic properties of the cerebrospinal fluid and of serum disappear. After ultrafiltration, as after dialysis, one does not observe the hypnotoxic property." (p 212) (Legendre and Piéron 1912a).

In 1912 also, Legendre and Piéron (1912b) published their first paper devoted to the effects of oxidation on serum. 'Panache' received, in the 4th ventricle at 39°C, serum from sleep deprived 'Castor' (see above) that had been treated for one hour with bubbling oxygen. This treatment induced clear-cut sleepiness and the usual cortical disturbances in the frontal cortex. (We will no longer repeat that, in each procedure, a corresponding volume of CSF was extracted from the recipient animal before administration). The same experiment was performed on 'Bull' after two hours of oxidation of 'Castor's' serum. The induced sleepiness was very light, and only rare frontal cells were shown to be disturbed. Then, the normal 'Maure' received sleep-deprived serum at 39°C from 'Robuste' after 2 h 10 min of oxidation. Inertia, but not clear-cut sleepiness, was observed. Frontal, crucial, and occipital neurons showed only rare chromatolysis. It should be recalled that 'Robuste' showed no strong sleep attempts even after long-term sleep deprivation. Next, 'Fez', another control, received sleep-deprived serum from 'Tunis' (see above) after 34 h oxidation at 39°C. There was no sleepiness. Finally, 'Madrid received serum from 'Tunis' that had been maintained at 15°C in the dark for 28 days. Madrid showed strong sleepiness and soon fell into a deep sleep. The occipital cortex cells were normal, the crucial area was nearly normal, and, in the frontal cortex, the large pyramidal and polymorph cells were very disturbed.

> "Thus, the hypnotoxic property, which is destroyed by oxidation, does not spontaneously disappear in darkness, even after four weeks" (p 275) (Legendre and Piéron 1912b).

Still in 1912, Legendre and Piéron (1912c) continued to characterize the properties of their 'hypnotoxin'. In 'Mina', serum from the sleep-deprived 'Robuste' that had been dried out with alcohol was dissolved in physiological water (distilled water with NaCl added to physiological levels) and introduced into the fourth ventricle. This treatment induced inertia, but not clear-cut sleepiness; there was also no histological deterioration. Similarly resuspended serum from 'Robuste' was injected into 'Domard'. This treatment induced a strong need for sleep, and frontal and cross area pyramidal and polymorph cells were very disturbed (chromatolysis, etc. ...); even occasional neurons in the occipital cortex showed the same disturbances. Then, 'Clignard' received the same injection as Mina, although in this case the serum was obtained from a sleep-deprived 'Castor'; the treatment induced a strong need for sleep. 'Galeux' also received alcohol-dehydrated serum that was later resuspended in physiological water, from 'Robuste'; in this case, the animal remained awake, without any histological deterioration. 'Resistant' and 'Lili' received a similar solution prepared from serum from the sleep-deprived 'Tunis'. While both animals showed a strong tendency to sleep, the histological analysis, undertaken only on 'Résistant', showed frontal cortex and, to a lesser extent, cross-level disturbances. Control experiments, using extracts from the non-sleep-deprived dogs 'Riquiqui', 'Fuyard', and 'Follepatte', did not show any induced sleepiness. "Thus, the phenomena of somnolence or of true sleep, with accompanying cellular alterations, are caused by the part of the serum that is insoluble in alcohol and that is soluble in distilled water...In sum, we can discuss the presence, in the blood, the cerebrospinal fluid, and the cerebral substance, in dogs subjected to prolonged sleep deprivation, of a 'hypnotoxin' that is probably a substance resulting from the decomposition of albuminoids during cerebral metabolism; this toxin is soluble in water, insoluble in alcohol, is destroyed by heating to 65°C or by prolonged oxidation, and is non-dialyzable; all of these are features that do not allow one to hope for its isolation at the moment" (p 304) (Legendre and Piéron 1912c).

Still in 1912, Toulouse and Piéron (1912) studied variations in patellar reflexes during sleep in humans. This work was an experimental study carried out according to the precise, well developed method that had been previously published by Piéron (1908i; 1810d). "The influence of sleep on the tendon reflexes has been the object of absolutely contradictory opinions ... We have also performed research with the goal of elucidating this point, using the sole correct method for studying reflexes, to determine the threshold of rotular reflex using our clinical reflexometer (Piéron, 1908b) ... The value of the threshold, that is, the weakest stimulation that is capable of provoking a contraction of the femoral quadriceps, is expressed by the angular height of the fall of the hammer onto the rotular tendon; the value shown in parentheses is the effect empirically determined using a spring, substituted for the tendon, and compressed by the hammer raised to the same angular height." (p 271). We provide here one example from all the results presented by the authors:

7.40 p.m. Lying 28° (320 gr)
Midnight. Asleep since 10 p.m.
Arousal during measurement 37° (455 gr)
3.10 a.m. Asleep, but arousal again 36° (440 gr)
6.10 a.m. Awakened 30° (350 gr)

> "The results show in the clearest possible way the depressive influence of sleep on the excitability reflex, an influence which is not due to the nocturnal phase of the circadian cycle, as it did not occur in the awake subject" (p 273) (Toulouse and Piéron 1912).

The authors then demonstrated, in several experiments performed on an epileptic patient, that bromide (at 2 and 4 gr daily) decreases reflexivity, as studied using Piéron's (1910d) methodology (see above). Indeed, the threshold of response was increased.

Finally, the year after, Legendre and Piéron (1913) wrote their last common paper on sleep that I was able to find. It was a long, detailed analysis and synthesis of all of their previously published results. They recount that in total, 13 dogs were sleep deprived for from 150 to 293 hours between 1906 to

1911, and that 48 injections of sleep-deprived or control serum, CSF, or brain extracts were performed, particularly into the 4th ventricle, into different dogs during this long-lasting research.

The authors concluded:

> "The results of this research show us that the hypnotic property developed during long periods of sleep deprivation is destroyed by heating to 65° for several minutes, that it is not susceptible to dialysis or to crossing the collodion membrane by ultrafiltration, that prolonged oxidation makes it disappear, and that it is found in the part of the serum that is insoluble in alcohol and soluble in distilled water; all of these properties are common to the diastases and to a large number of toxins ... A prolonged waking state produces in the organism, probably as a waste product of cerebral metabolism, the formation of a toxin that causes local cellular lesions and a pressing need for sleep, phenomena which are obviously related ... The normal destruction of this waste product, of this toxin, must undoubtedly be achieved by an oxidation mechanism during sleep ... Hence, during experimentally induced sleep deprivation, there is a dangerous, or even mortal, accumulation...when hypnic rest does not intervene to stop this excessive production and to allow anti-toxic and repairing processes to restore the cerebral cells to a normal functional state." (p 260-261) (Legendre and Piéron 1913).

Also in 1913, and therefore following the defense of his doctoral dissertation, Piéron (1913b) published an article providing a broad overview of sleep. To begin, he reviewed sleep processes in the animal kingdom, displaying a beautiful knowledge of immobility and true sleep in invertebrates and vertebrates, and referring to pseudo-sleep in some species. He summarized his observations by concluding: "In sum, sleep involving the temporary and almost complete interruption of sensorimotor relations of a being with its environment is not a universal biological phenomenon." (p 291). Then, he analyzed sleep in humans and characterized it (prior to any electrophysiological knowledge) as "a great increase in excitability thresholds ... and ... an almost complete absence of spontaneous activity, with a very general decrease in muscular tonus." (p 291). In this part of the article, he also recalled the different pathological causes of sleep (anemia, oxygen deprivation, brain compression, tumors, trypanosomiasis, etc.). In a new paragraph, he considered hibernation: "The real question of hibernation is the renunciation by the organism of the maintenance of its thermic level ... Hibernal torpor has nothing in common with true sleep." (p 292). The next section was devoted to sleep factors, in which he first describes his method of sleep deprivation to create a pressure for sleep. Then, he detailed the induced histological disturbances, and the causal relationship between the sleep factor and the histological disturbances. He recalled that the 'hypnotoxin' is destroyed by heat and by oxidation, that it is soluble in water, and that it is found in the part of the serum that can be precipitated by alcohol. "It appears to be similar to properties of diastases ... and seems linked to the disintegration of cerebral albuminoids, being present in the cerebrospinal fluid." (p 295). Afterwards, Piéron reviewed various theories of sleep, and postulated "a two-fold mechanism of sleep, a deep, fundamental mechanism, which is the toxic mechanism, and a supplementary mechanism, which is more fragile, an inhibitory mechanism that anticipates the true cause." (p 296). In the final part of the article, he emphasizes the notion of anticipation in biology in general, and in sleep generation more specifically. In the same way that "the animal breathes without waiting for carbonic acid to accumulate, there must have been an anticipation, a reaction to very low levels, and then a rhythmization .., In the same way, the suppression of cerebral functions is bought about by the accumulation of toxic waste products; this suspension was able to occur with minimal levels of waste product and to rhythmize, to recur periodically ... The cerebral intoxication would play the role of providing a protective mechanism that leads to a suspension of function, in the course of which the toxic waste products, present at minimal levels, could be oxidized." (p 296). To conclude, he states: "The problem of sleep is obviously very complex; but we have a solid experimental handhold on the hypnotoxic phenomena brought about by prolonged sleep deprivation, a foothold that allows us to find our footing amidst an ocean of theories and hypotheses." (p 298) (Piéron 1913b).

A commentary was written much later by Piéron (1927). This commentary concerned a discussion about a report by J. Lhermitte and A. Tournay (1927) on normal and pathological sleep that took place at the French neurological society. Piéron noted the progress that had been made in studies devoted to the psychogalvanic reflex that occurs during sleep, i.e., the observed increased skin resistance. He recalled his research on the 'hypnotoxin': "There does not seem to be, in the initial stages (of tiredness), a progressive intoxication that leads to normal sleep. It is an inhibitory defense reaction against this intoxication that leads to normal sleep, and we can speak of an instinct… as with diverse activities of vegetative life. Respiratory activities, or activities resulting from hunger, give us analogous examples of anticipation" (p 831). "In the case of narcolepsy, are there not cases where a metabolic problem leads to the more rapid and intense production of the hypnotoxin? Research into a toxic activity of this type in the CSF of such patients would be quite desirable" (p 832) (Piéron 1927).

Piéron (1952) published a final, very original paper about sleep. It was related to his personal observation that, during light sleep, the perception and integration of the ringing of his pendulum clock is disturbed.

> "Hearing the tonal component of the strikes on the chime, when the pendulum rings the hour, is completely lacking as long as awakening has not occurred, but can be abruptly restored, in less than a second, in the interval between two strikes, with its proper characteristics, and its prolongation by resonance of the vibrating chime, as soon as waking up occurs ..."
>
> ... During light sleep, what is heard, without being interpreted, is the brief sound of the hammer hitting the chime ... in no case is the sound-based stimulation integrated into a dream, but they provoke awakening, which allows the experience to be integrated into vigilant thought...
>
> ... From what comes the dissociation of tonal hearing, during the course of an incomplete hypnic interruption of auditory sensitivity? ... The most probable hypothesis is that of a cortical dissociation. A double auditory projection has been demonstrated in the cortex of mammals ...: a surface close to the tactile sphere was responsive, even after the destruction of the classical zones of auditory projection ... which clearly distinguishes it from secondary zones that are most likely perceptive...In this zone, there is no clear pattern of localization as a function of the strength of the sound ... unlike the zone of the principal projection, where the tonal localization was established ... it is thus tempting to attribute to such a receptive zone the responsibility of a crude atonal response, of a primitive nature, that could be more resistant to the hypnic inhibition of exteroceptive sensation, less fragile than the zone of the delicate tonal responses." (p 394-395) (Piéron1952).

It has to be underlined that this paper was published one year prior to the discovery of rapid eye movement (REM) sleep by Aserinsky and Kleitman (1953a,b). Consequently, light sleep has to be understood as sleep onset and/or slow wave sleep (mainly stage II).

Chapter 4

Conclusion

Piéron's work on immobility in lower species as a possible indicator of sleep (Piéron, 1908d; 1910e), as well as on true sleep in mammals, was very original in the beginning of the last century, particularly in the absence of any information about electrophysiology. Although part of his research on temperature regulation was essentially the attentive replication and deepening of previous studies (Toulouse and Piéron 1906a,b,c, 1907a,b), the great majority of it was directed to new topics. It was the first time that the consequences of sleep deprivation (without any physical fatigue) on brain state was explored, showing particularly that the abnormalities of nerve cells, essentially localized in the phylogenetically most recent frontal cortex, are reversed by recovery of sleep. In relation to sleep mechanisms, the idea of exploring the possible influence of a sleep factor of a chemical nature was original at that time, although the concept of auto-intoxication, which was later hypothesized in particular to be related to carbonic acid and deficits in oxygen, had already been advanced (Durham 1860). To study it by transfer of biological products was applied for the first time, and became usual for many later researchers. The experimental method he used was very carefully developed, involving multiple progressive steps and the transfer of blood (serum), brain, and CSF extracts. The attentive successive steps to characterize the chemical properties of the sleep factor identifiable in those days are also to be underlined. Perhaps because he was originally a psychologist, he did not have the idea of directly testing CSF from sleep-deprived animals by icv injection. However, it is true that Ishimori (1909), working in the same period, also only succeeded in subcutaneously injecting brain extracts at the abdominal level. Ishimori's first experiment regarding sleep deprivation was of a shorter duration than Piéron's, lasting for up to 113 hours. This experiment was also performed in young dogs, and its results, involving the induction of sleepiness in normal dogs, were obtained in March-April 1907.

It was the same year that Legendre and Piéron (1907a,b) and Piéron (1907d) published their first biological and histological descriptions of the consequences of long-duration sleep deprivation, as well as their method for the study of sleep factors. However, the observation of the sleep-inducing effects of brain extracts was first published in 1910, in Japanese, by Ishimori (1909). As stated by Kubota (1989), "unfortunately, his contribution to the field of sleep research had been virtually forgotten until his paper… was found by K. Uchizono" (1984) (quoted by Kubota). It must be mentioned that, in Eastern countries, Legendre and Piéron's experiment on sleep-inducing factors was later reproduced in dogs (Ivy and Schnedorf, 1937; Schnedorf and Ivy, 1939), but these later experiments also showed that these factors, like normal ventricular liquid, increases the body temperature, which by itself induces sleepiness. Thus, "the normal picture of sleep is not produced" (p 504) (Schnedorf and Ivy, 1939). Moreover, two previous clinical observations had already shown that increased body temperature favors sleep (Lindig, 1922; Lust, 1921). As noted by Kubota, the later clear confirmation of such a sleep-inducing substance ("Factor S") was provided by Pappenheimer's team, using CSF and brainstem-cortex extracts from sleep-deprived ruminants (goats and sheep); these extracts were icv injected into rodents (rats and rabbits), inducing sleepiness and slow wave EEG sleep activity {Pappenheimer et al., 1975). Several subsequent studies have further enriched our knowledge on this topic (Garcia-Garcia et al., 2009).

It seems impossible to summarize the extraordinarily large body of sleep-related knowledge and associated literature that is concentrated in *Le problème physiologique du sommeil*. The definition of sleep that he formulated in his book, coming at the end of his work on sleep, was: "a periodically necessary state, occurring with a periodicity that is relatively independent of exterior circumstances, and characterized by the suspension of the complex sensorimotor relationships that unite the being with its environment and allow the continuation of its life, in particular through feeding." (p 3). This definition is in good accordance with the sleep-related knowledge that was available at the time. Indeed, already in 1882, Duval had written that "normal sleep is one of the forms of the law of functional periodicity, a law which has its reason for existence in the necessity of repairing materials that are constantly being worn out by the state of activity, the repair of which cannot be sufficiently accomplished during the continuity of the action of the organ." (p 273) … and also “A state of suspension of relationship functions” (p 265) with the maintenance of digestion. (Duval 1882). The different parts of Piéron’s thesis were first devoted to an analysis of the numerous physiological concomitants of sleep found in the literature, with its circulatory, respiratory, and digestive aspects, complemented by data related to thermogenesis and sensorimotor phenomena. He then analyzed various states that are behaviorally analogous to sleep, particularly comatose states, narcolepsy, lethargy, forms of sleepiness, and then narcosis and hypnosis, and hibernation; he also included a few pages on normal sleep and sleep states. The third part concerns the experimental problem of sleep factors and was primarily devoted to a description of his own results. The fourth part concerns different theories of sleep, and the last section presents a final discussion of the different aspects of the physiological problem of sleep. This monumental work, once again, comprised 1,229 bibliographic references.

Later, in 1950, Piéron became the first president of the International Union of Scientific Psychology. Throughout his scientific life, he was highly active, and in the last twelve years of his life he published: the remarkable *Vocabulaire de psychologie*, 1953 Presses Universitaire de France (PUF); *La psychophysique*, and *Les besoins* (“Needs”), 1953, in the *Traité de psychologie expérimentale*, (PUF); *Le Traité de psychologie appliquée*, volumes I to VII, 1955-56 (PUF); *“L’information*”, 1957, in *Encyclopédie française; De l’actinie à l’Homme*, 1959 ("From Anemones to Man", 2 vol., PUF); *La sensation,* 1960 (PUF); *La vision en lumière intermitente,* 1961 ("Vision in intermittent light"), CNRS; *Examens et docimologie*, 1963 (PUF). As stated by Littman (1971), these publications showed “the very diversity of his research interests” (p 204).

An interesting point that highlights the scientific reasoning that guided Piéron throughout his career was that he attributed the study of consciousness only to philosophers, while in his own approach to psychology he exclusively explored the physiological basis of behavior; according to Chauchard, it was “excessive [of him] to refuse to recognize that it is precisely the cerebral mechanisms of consciousness that neurophysiology is beginning to elucidate.” (p 6927) (Chauchard 1964). This remark is even more valid today, with the remarkable development that has taken place in neuro- and psychopharmacological studies and imaging techniques. Recent results show that linguistic processing and social communication occur 3 months before term (Mahmoudzadeh et al. 2013).

To conclude, Paul Fraisse, Piéron’s successor at the head of the Institut de Psychologie, wrote in 1965: "No psychologist will later be able to have the quasi universality of a Henry Piéron. Our science is so developed now that each individual must choose his own specific path. But for all of us, Henri Piéron leaves us a body of teaching and an example". (p 4) (Fraisse, 1965).

Henri Piéron died on November 6, 1964.

Nathaniel Kleitman

Chapter 5

Nathaniel Kleitman

Nathaniel Kleitman was born in 1895 in Kishinev (Russia) and was 20 years old when he emigrated to the United States. He became a naturalized citizen in 1918. He obtained his BSc degree at the City College of New York in 1919, and his M.A. at Columbia University in 1920. After working as an instructor in physiology and pharmacology at the University of Georgia, he completed his PhD in physiology at Chicago University, finishing *summa cum laude* in 1923. He founded his sleep research laboratory at the same university in 1925-26, and worked there throughout his career. He taught until 1960, when he retired (Dement, 2001). (Figure 2).

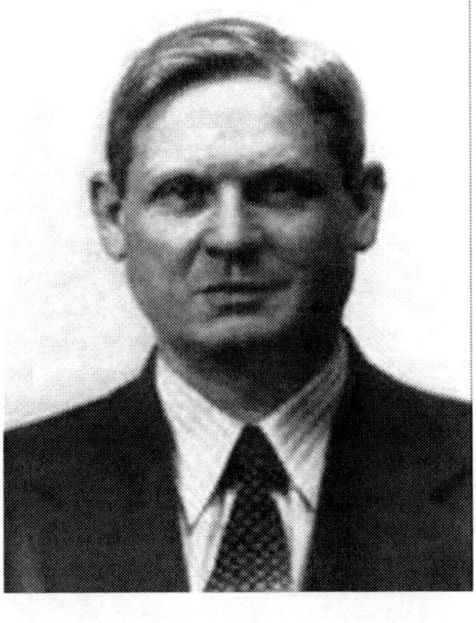

Figure 2. Nathaniel Kleitman. Reprinted from *Archives Italiennes de Biologie*.

As will be seen, his knowledge of sleep literature was vast, and while he stated "my own ability is limited to French, German, Italian and Russian, I was fortunate in securing the assistance of B.B. Lifschultz, whose knowledge of the Scandinavian languages, as well as of Dutch and Spanish, was of invaluable help to me in gathering and classifying the bibliographical material" (p ix) (Kleitman, 1939).

Chapter 6

Sleep Knowledge at the Period Between Pieron's Final Work and the Beginning of Kleitman's Research

The main element defining this period was the dramatic appearance of encephalitis lethargica, which killed even more Europeans than WWI. Constantin von Economo is regarded as the definitive author concerning this epidemic (Economo 1917), although Cruchet et al. (1917) made similar initial clinical observations. Economo beautifully discovered that fatal sleepiness was correlated with posterior hypothalamic lesions, whereas fatal excitement was related to anterior hypothalamic lesions (Economo 1928, Khatami et al. 2012). It is of interest that animal research confirmed these observations only much later on during Kleitman's career: Ranson (1939), Nauta (1946) Manceau and Jorda (1948), McGinty (1969) and others for induced sleepiness by posterior hypothalamic lesions; Hess (1931), Hess jr, Akert and Koella (1950) Sterman and Clemente (1962) and others for sleep induced by anterior hypothalamic stimulation (Hess 2012); and Manceau and Jorda (1948), Maire and Patton (1954), McGinty and Sterman (1968) and others for hyperarousal induced by lesions at the same location. For details see Gottesmann (2001).

Chapter 7

Kleitman's Research

His first paper on sleep (Kleitman, 1923) appeared when he was 28. It is of high interest to show its first page, since it is very informative (Figure 3).

First, it is telling for both the plural main title and for the "I" that precedes the sub-title; Kleitman's intention was clearly to work on the same sleep topic on a long-term basis. Second, he is the sole author of the research and, although at the end of the paper he thanks several individuals for their help, the decision to undertake the study of sleep seems to have been his own. Third, all of the sentences of the first paragraph could still be encountered in the Introductions of many modern papers (!). Finally, in the second paragraph, he honors the work of Henri Piéron, as he did later in his two editions of *Sleep and Wakefulness* (1939, 1963).

As the title indicates, the paper was devoted to the study of the consequences of prolonged sleep deprivation. In contrast to Piéron's sleep deprivation study, which was performed on dogs and which sought to identify the chemical basis of the imperative need for sleep, Kleitman's research first involved students who were deprived for from 40 to 115 hours, with the goal of analyzing the potential modification of several biological parameters; his research was thus rather devoted to the consequences of sleep deprivation.

> "The only method that was found to work consisted in having the subject keep moving throughout the night, with short periods of rest sitting down ... For the determination of pulse, temperature, respiratory rate and blood pressure, the subject was allowed to lie completely relaxed for at least 15 minutes, and in measuring basal metabolism, for at least 30 minutes … All the determinations were made daily at 7 a.m." (p 69).

STUDIES ON THE PHYSIOLOGY OF SLEEP

I. The Effects of Prolonged Sleeplessness on Man

NATHANIEL KLEITMAN

From the Hull Physiological Laboratory of the University of Chicago

Received for publication May 28, 1923

Most investigators of the physiology of sleep, in reporting their findings, remind their readers, by way of apology, of the tremendous importance of the subject for the advancement of our knowledge of physiology as a science, as well as for the rational treatment of insomnia. They also like to record the fact that the average individual spends more than a third of his life in sleep, has been doing this from time immemorial, and raise the question whether eight hours or more of sleep a day really constitutes the minimum penalty for keeping awake the rest of the time. It seems reasonable to suspect that as in the case of protein consumption, there is a large "factor of safety" in the amount of sleep we are getting, and that it could be considerably reduced without impairment of health or loss of efficiency. This and other questions related to industrial physiology, especially physiology of fatigue, can be answered only by a thorough systematic study of the subject. But curiously enough, there are scarcely a dozen investigators engaged at any one time in the study of this great physiological mystery, and most of these workers are psychologists. It seems that because animals are not very well adapted for this work and the human beings that are available cannot be dissected, physiologists have allowed the psychologists to tackle this problem as best they could.

In this paper references will be made to both physiological and psychological literature. One of the best books ever written on the subject of sleep is Piéron's *Le Problème Physiologique du Sommeil* (1), which besides embodying the results of original research on sleep from the histological, biochemical and physiological standpoints (this by a psychologist!) contains a valuable and exhaustive bibliography brought up to 1912. To save space references will be given only to those papers which appeared after 1912, or have not been included in Piéron's bibliography; others referred to as (P) will be found in Piéron's bibliography.

Figure 3. Introduction of Kleitman's first sleep paper. Reprinted from *American Journal of Physiology*.

Further to the above described methodology (point '1.'), Kleitman's exceptional extended summary of the paper best expresses the obtained results:

> "2. Subjectively the persons employed could easily keep awake while engaged in some sort of activity, but felt very drowsy when sitting, and fell asleep immediately on lying down.
>
> 3. Muscular relaxation induces sleep under normal conditions ... but practically precipitates sleep under conditions of experimental insomnia.
>
> 4. Blood sugar, alkaline reserve of the blood and plasma, percentage of hemoglobin, percentage of corpuscles, red and white blood cell count, body weight, basal metabolic rate, appetite, temperature, ability to name letters and to do arithmetic, all of these showed no variations from normal during the period of sleeplessness.
>
> 5. Respiration, heart rate, blood pressure showed a marked decrease in insomnia, but this decrease was mainly due to greater muscular relaxation in the sleepy subject.
>
> 6. Numerous reflexes were found to be present in sleep following insomnia, but the response was somewhat sluggish. Sleep seemed to be deeper six hours after its onset than at the end of two hours.
>
> 7. A positive Babinski reflex could be elicited in every subject tested during the sleep that followed insomnia. It is interpreted as indicating a functional block of the pyramidal system of fibers.
>
> 8. This reflex could be reversed by rapidly repeated stimulation of the sole. The depth of the sleep decreased at the same time. This indicates that a number of subliminal stimuli overcome the synaptic resistance and produce a flexion of the great toe.
>
> 9. There is a greater excretion of phosphates and acids at night; but on reverse routine, when the subject sleeping in the daytime, this condition is reversed, indicating that the increased excretion is due to sleep.
>
> 10. There is a greater excretion of chlorides in the daytime; the same is true in insomnia; but there is a tendency to reversal in the subject that sleeps during the day.
>
> 11. The excretion of total nitrogen and of creatinine shows little diurnal variation, and is unaffected by either insomnia or reversed routine.
>
> 12. There is some evidence that the diurnal temperature variation is due to the alternation of sleep and wakefulness, and the temperature wave tends to be effaced during prolonged insomnia.
>
> 13. The onset of sleep is probably due to complete muscular relaxation, voluntary or involuntary.
>
> 14. A provisional theory is proposed based on the conception of "levels" in the central nervous system, as first elaborated by Hughlings

> Jackson. Sleep may be due to fatigue of the highest centers of consciousness, and dreaming to the persistence of the activity of the lower centers" (p 91).

To complete the last point concerning Hughlings Jackson, Kleitman quoted him as follows: "the most complex nervous arrangements, centers and levels are the least organized; the simple, the most organized." Kleitman added: "In our experiments … the only definite effect of insomnia was the depression of the activity of the highest centers that are concerned in analyzing sensations and in solving problems. All our subjects found that they could not study after one night of wakefulness, although they could do ordinary routine laboratory work fairly successfully throughout the entire period of insomnia. The temporary dissociation of consciousness observed in N.K. (certainly Nathaniel Kleitman since he was often subject in the experiments)… points in the same direction ... On the histological side Piéron reports that he found definitely localized changes in the brain of dogs killed after prolonged periods of sleeplessness, and he indicates that these higher levels have definite localizations in the cortex." (p 87-88).

With respect to dreaming, Kleitman discussed the 'low integration level' of external and internal stimuli. "The literature of the subject is full of accounts of how a trivial external happening was misinterpreted by the dreamer and a curious dream built around it ... The switching off' of the pyramidal tracts which give rise to the positive Babinski prevents the efferent impulses from reaching the muscles and thereby protects the sleeper from being aroused by the powerful proprioceptive impulses that should in such event be sent up from the muscles. Sleepwalkers apparently lack the ability to completely shunt off the pyramidal tracts … and their dreams give rise to actual movements" (p 89).

The final sentence of Kleitman's conclusion was the following quotation from Piéron: "Une théorie n'est pas la solution d'un problème, c'est (au) contraire l'énoncé d'un problème à résoudre" ("A theory is not the solution to a problem, it's in contrast the enunciation of a problem to be solved.") (p 90) (Kleitman 1923).

In 1923, Kleitman published another paper devoted to the consequences of long-term sleep deprivation in which he appeared as second author (Lee and Kleitman 1923). "The purpose … was to determine if any changes occur in the activity of higher and lower centers of the nervous system." (p 141). The experiment was performed on one subject "who underwent six (?) sleepless periods, three of 60 hours, two of 90 hours and two of 114 hours, separated by long control periods" (p 141). The knee-jerk reflex was first studied using a method that was more sophisticated than that of Piéron (1910c,d), and then the pupillary reflex was examined. In addition, the authors evaluated the sensory threshold for faradic stimuli, steadiness as measured using a device fixed on the head which had been described in the literature, and reaction time, and they also asked the subjects to perform certain tasks: naming of opposites, naming colors, cancelation in printed lists, and mental arithmetic. The results first showed that "the knee-jerk is not affected by insomnia, but promptly disappears with the onset of sleep (Figure 4).

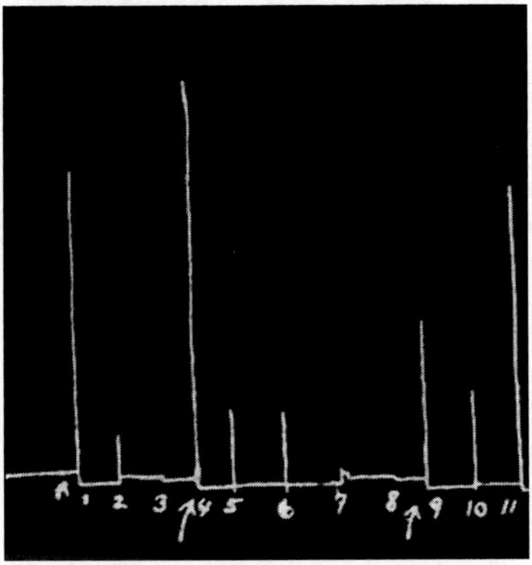

Figure 4. Knee-jerk variation during sleep deprivation. "Although knee-jerks varied from day to day in our control periods, albeit only within definite limits … no changes whatsoever could be observed … as a result of sleeplessness … Another interesting result was the complete disappearance (of the response) … if the subject happened to fall asleep during the test" (p 147). Arrows: waking. Reprinted from *American Journal of Physiology*.

> … The pupillary reflex persists practically unchanged during insomnia, but in dim lights of standard intensity, the diameter of the pupil is much smaller than normal. The sensory threshold of faradic stimuli, the ability to react to auditory and visual stimuli, to name opposites, to multiply mentally, all these show no change in insomnia (confirming data of literature). The ability to name colors was not impaired during insomnia, if the number of colors was small (100), but when the subject had to name 1200 colors in succession, he spent more time and made more errors than during the control periods, thus showing inability to

sustain attention under these conditions. (Finally) the power to maintain one's equilibrium, applying the graphic method ... showed marked deterioration during insomnia, but this was possibly due to concomitant muscular fatigue" (p 151) (Lee and Kleitman 1923) (Figure 5).

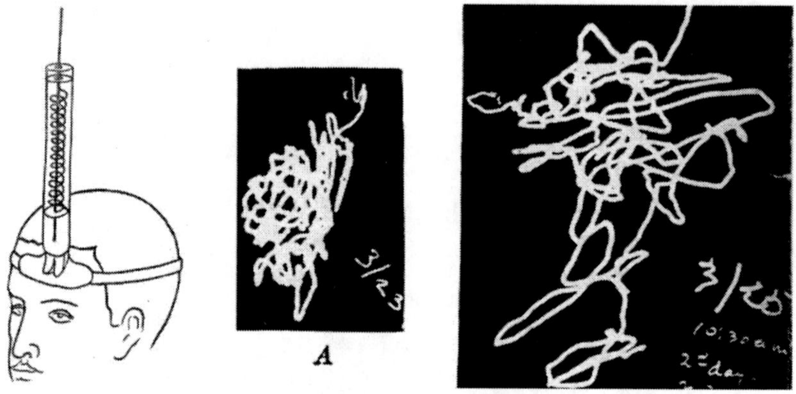

Figure 5. Disturbances in steadiness during sleep deprivation. On the left, a sketch of the device. "The wire allowed recording of the swinging of the body by lowering a horizontal metal plate covered with smoked paper until the paper touched the tip of the wire. The fine spring which carried the wire insured continuous contact between the wire and the smoked surface, with a minimum of friction. The recording was entirely inaudible" (p 145). On the right, A: before sleep deprivation, B: after sleep deprivation (duration not indicated). Reprinted from *American Journal of Physiology*.

At the end of the year 1923 the results already show the significant progression of ideas and techniques in comparison with Piéron's time.

The next paper, published by Kleitman (1925), aimed to extend a result obtained in the previous paper which had shown an increase in urine phosphates and acid elimination during the night, suggesting that it was related to sleep.

"For a long time it was believed that mental activity had an influence on phosphorus metabolism, and numerous experiments were undertaken to determine the effect of intellectual work on the elimination of phosphorus in the urine. The various investigators were especially interested in determining the effect of sleep on the excretion of phosphorus in the urine, since sleep is a period of minimal activity ... Aside from the decrease of mental activity during sleep, there is also present a more or less complete relaxation of the body musculature. We

> decided to investigate these two phases (waking and sleep) separately. In one instance we followed the phosphorus elimination in sleep and wakefulness for many weeks as a normal control, and after this, during a period of presumably decreased mental activity resulting from the daily administration of comparatively large doses of potassium bromide. To study the effect of muscular relaxation, we analyzed the urine secreted during short periodical strenuous muscular work, and that secreted during like periods before and after the exercise." (p 225-226)

The results showed that the urine secreted during sleep contained much more phosphorus than that observed during waking. In addition, the acid level was also increased. This finding confirmed results that had previously been obtained both by Kleitman's group and by other researchers. The administration of potassium bromide did not affect the results,

> "indicating that mental activity hardly played a part in determining this lesser excretion of phosphorus during waking ... That there is a parallelism between the rate of excretion of phosphorus and that of acid had been noticed by all observers. The question has been often asked whether the phosphate excretion followed that of acid, or whether the acidity of the urine was determined by the amount of phosphorus excreted". (p 233).

In this paper, Kleitman showed that this parallelism is not always obvious and that during exercise, phosphorus excretion is massively decreased while acidity is unchanged, and that during consecutive relaxation a higher amount of phosphorus is released.

> "It seems probable that during the exercise some phosphorus is taken up by the muscle, and therefore not all the phosphorus catabolized is excreted by the kidneys ... (He concluded) "It seems that phosphorus is in no way related to the mechanism of sleep as such, but is merely a concomitant of sleep, depending directly upon complete muscular relaxation." (236-237) (Kleitman 1925).

Reed and Kleitman (1926) studied the effects of sleep on respiration. Nine healthy adult subjects (including two women) underwent an experimental procedure principally composed of "two sensitive pneumographs placed, one high around the subject's chest, the other around the abdomen at about the level of umbilicus." (p 601).

"The respiratory rate was frequently increased on passing from wakefulness to sound sleep, although in nearly as many cases there was no change in rate. Very slow normal rates were always increased. If the respiration was even and regular while awake, it usually became progressively less regular during somnolence, but became regular again in sound sleep. If respiration was irregular in the beginning, this irregularity generally persisted throughout somnolence, sometimes becoming more pronounced, but generally disappearing during deep sleep. The irregularity in respiration was commonly aperiodic, but it sometimes assumed a definite periodicity, resembling Cheyne-Stokes breathing. While changes in the thoracic and abdominal movements were ordinarily the same, pronounced irregularity sometimes occurred in one of these movements alone …

… The so-called inversion of the ratio between the thoracic and abdominal amplitudes on going to sleep did not take place. In the majority of experiments the amplitude of the abdominal excursions was absolutely decreased on going to sleep, and in a number of experiments the amplitude of the thoracic excursions was absolutely increased. The position occupied by the subject during the experiment did not seem to influence the direction of the changes occurring …

… A subliminal auditory stimulus that failed to elicit a response from the subject was frequently sufficient to produce some modification of respiration …

… The changes observed were not always the same in a given subject in successive experiments, nor even in the same test on being awakened and allowed to fall asleep again." (p 608) (Reed and Kleitman 1926).

In 1927 Kleitman (1927) working alone, published a new paper on sleep deprivation. For the first time, this research was performed not in humans, but in puppies.

"The tests to be described here were made in 1923, at the same time that similar experiments were performed in human beings. The brains and other parts of the nervous system of experimental and control animals were removed at the moment of death and preserved for detailed histologic examination. No one competent to prepare this material was available at that time, and the results of the experiments remained unpublished. The neurological data have recently been obtained." (p 386).

Kleitman first recounted the sleep deprivation method used by Piéron (see above) and its behavioral consequences. "Our dogs, however, managed to sleep very well while hanging on the chain, but we found walking to be an excellent method of keeping them awake. We therefore adopted the simple method of watching the animals constantly, tugging them by the chain when they were about to fall asleep, walking them a little when tugging was not effective... To avoid the necessity of carrying on an experiment for more than a few days we used puppies whose need for sleep is much more acute than that of adult dogs." (p 386). Their ages varied from six weeks to three months. Each sleep-deprived puppy was coupled to a control. If the puppy was killed at the end of an experiment, or spontaneously died, the control puppy was killed at the same time and an autopsy performed on both, with brain and spinal cord being removed and preserved. The author carefully described the behavior of the deprived puppies for two to seven days: progressive loss of interest in its surroundings, photophobia, sometimes "the transformation of a sleepy apathetic creature into an alert and widely awake animal ... As a rule, the approaching end was characterized by a gradually increasing muscular weakness, the animals standing or walking in a peculiar manner: their front paws would flex anteriorly giving them an appearance of being 'flat-footed'. At such times the puppies showed disturbances in body righting." (p 388). When allowed to, or during recovery, they were able to sleep in a vertical position, with head downward, held in the air by one foot.

Table 5. Blood study during sleep deprivation in puppies

A comparison between the red blood cell count of a puppy deprived of sleep for several days (W) and that of its litter mate that was allowed to sleep ad libitum (S)

DATE	R.B.C. IN THOUSANDS PER CUBIC MILIMETER		DATE	R.B.C. IN THOUSANDS PER CUBIC MILIMETER	
	W	S		W	S
February 17	4480	4580	March 3	4880	4330
18	*4860*	4640	4	4480	4320
19	*4320*	4450	7	4680	4650
21	*3440*	4640	10	4910	4480
22	*3800*	4520	13	*4816*	4620
25	4220	4590	14	*4724*	4768
26	4460	4640	15	*4100*	4590
28	3928	4860	16	*3920*	4670
			17	*4080*	4672
			18	*3370*	4652
			19	*3520*	4900

Biological results showed that there was nearly no change in body weight, temperature, heart or respiratory rate, nor were there alterations in blood sugar, blood albumin levels, hemoglobin, or white blood cells. "The only marked change noted was in the red blood cell account, which fell appreciably, sometimes more than 25 per cent, in the experimental animals (Table 5). The results of a neurological study of the various parts of the central nervous system were entirely negative." (p 389-390).

It is interesting to note that Kleitman's observation that dogs were able to sleep even while hanging on the chain explains why it was possible for Piéron's dogs to be deprived for much longer durations without inducing death, than the deprivation performed by Manaceine (1894) (Kovalzon 2012).

In the second part of the paper, Kleitman made several observations regarding normal sleep in the puppies which complemented conclusions made by previous researchers. He confirmed that when the puppies were immobilized in a dorsal position, after a while they were able to begin to sleep, often after a yawn or two. "Once on sleep the puppies could be manipulated considerably without waking them up... Yawning was also a frequent accompaniment of awakening ... The most prominent feature of awakening, however, was the stiffening of the abdominal musculature which rendered the anterior abdominal wall taut." (p 391).

Then, under ether anesthesia and following a careful procedure, Kleitman removed part of the frontal and parietal bones on one side of the cranium to observe the brain. "No changes, either in the caliber of the blood vessels or in the general appearance of the brain could be detected when the puppy was passing from wakefulness to sleep, or back from sleep to the waking state. That was also the case when the puppies fell asleep spontaneously." (p 391-392).

> "In general, the results of these experiments are in support of the working hypothesis … that sleep comes from a decrease in the number of afferent impulses reaching the central nervous system from the sensorium, and that muscular relaxation, decreasing considerably the number of proprioceptive impulses, constitutes the last stage of the process by which sleep is precipitated." (p 394) (Kleitman 1927).

Kleitman (1929) published an impressive review entitled "Sleep". This 41-page paper (!) analyzed all of the findings available at the time, with one significant limitation: "In his monumental work on sleep published in 1913 Piéron covered critically and exhaustively the literature on the physiology and pathology of sleep. A good deal of information found in that book has become common knowledge by this time. For this reason I shall limit my review almost exclusively to papers that appeared after 1913." (p 624). There were only three exceptions, including Mauthner (1890), which had been previously cited by Piéron. In spite of this self-imposed limitation with respect to the years covered by his review, there were still 137 references cited for this short period 1913-1929!

As early as on the first page a definition of sleep is tentatively given, providing three properties:

> "1, a loss of critical reactivity to events in one's environment; 2, an increased threshold of general sensibility and reflex irritability; and 3, an ability of being aroused or brought back to the state of wakefulness. The term of sleep as used in this review will refer to ordinary diurnal sleep, short day naps and similar conditions resembling normal sleep and fulfilling the above mentioned three requirements. It will exclude hypnosis, narcosis and coma." (p 624).

Kleitman carefully analyzed all the available results and literature related to 1/ the phenomena that accompany sleep; 2/ The phenomena that precede sleep ; 3/ The phenomena that follow sleep; 4/ The effects of experimental abstention from sleep; 5/ Diseased conditions where sleep or its disturbances are among the prominent symptoms. 6/ Pharmacological agents producing sleep or sleep-like states. 7/ Theories of sleep. It is not possible here to analyze and summarize all of the described results and theories, except for Kleitman's theory of sleep, which is described above (Kleitman, 1923).

> "I do not … claim exclusive authorship of the ideas presented. Aside from the results of my experiments, the writings of (seven mentioned authors) and others suggested this scheme developed." (p 654).

The following ideas were successively detailed:

> "1/ Sleep is an easily reversible inactivity of the highest functional centers of the cerebral cortex. 2/ The inactivity is due to a functional break between the cerebral cortex and the other parts of the nervous system. 3/ The functional break results from a marked decrease in the number of afferent impulses from the sensorium, especially proprioceptive impulses which depend upon the degree of muscle tonus maintained. 4/ Sleep is due to fatigue of the neuromuscular mechanism concerned in the maintenance of muscular tonus. 5/ In the absence of such fatigue, sleep may result from complete muscular relaxation, intentional or unintentional. 6/ Diurnal alternation of wakefulness and sleep is a 'conditioned' phenomenon." (p 654-655).

In this discussion, it is useful to highlight Kleitman's comments on dreaming (since with Aserinsky (Aserinsky and Kleitman, 1953b), he later discovered rapid eye movement (REM) sleep, during which dreaming essentially appears).

> "To sleep, perchance to dream', is something to look forward to when one is not pressed for time. There is a general agreement that deep sleep is dreamless, and that we are more likely to dream just before awakening in the morning ... Subjective observations show that the main characteristic of a dream is a lack of critical analysis of its content … and (confirming other authors) the low integration of dreams as contrasted with the high integration of consciousness … and the abolition of the learning process ... It is evident that dreaming often starts as a result of afferent stimuli, extero- or interoceptive in character -- generally grossly misinterpreted -- but whether that is invariably the case is not known. The dreamer frequently wakes up in the course of a dream, but even before that happens the sleep become disturbed." (p 636-637).

Kleitman concluded the review as follows:

> "The problem of sleep has yet to be solved. There are many questions to be answered, some of them by repeating the work of individual observers. There is no authority but that of facts, and until isolated observations have been repeatedly confirmed they cannot be classed as established facts." (p 659) (Kleitman 1929).

In 1930, Kleitman (1930) published a short paper on the evolution of the conditioned salivary reflex during sleep. It fact, this was the application to sleep of other research (Kleitman and Crisler, 1927) that is absent from the references of both editions of Sleep and Wakefulness. Indeed, this reference does not concern sleep but is rather exclusively devoted to the conditioning of the salivary reflex, highlighting the very wide range of interests of the author.

> "In the usual scheme of experimentation on conditioned reflexes the application of the conditioned stimulus is always discontinued when, or before, the unconditioned stimulation begins. In the morphine-induced conditioned salivation studied in our laboratory (Kleitman and Crisler, 1927), this is not the case. The dogs used had permanent fistulae of the duct of one of the submaxillary glands, and this permitted the study of the salivary response quantitatively. They were placed in stands, mainly to insure the proper collection of saliva, and they remained in these stands throughout the entire test. A definite constant time after the dog was

placed in the stand he was given a subcutaneous injection of morphine. Repetition of this procedure once a day for several days resulted in a conditioned salivation becoming gradually established, the animal salivating on being placed in the stand, before the injection of morphine ... The average duration of the salivary flow after the injection (30 mg) varied from 15 to 20 minutes in different dogs (p 215) ...

... A particularity exhibited by this dog (the results describe only those obtained in a female) was a tendency to fall asleep while in the stand, both before the injection of morphine and after the effect of the injection were off ... As drowsiness appeared, the secretion generally diminished, and with the onset of sleep it would stop altogether. Waking the dog resulted in a flare-up of the salivary flow (p 217) (Figure 6).

... The behavior of this dog is not in agreement with the postulates of Pavlov's (1954) theory of sleep ... Sleep observed during the work on conditioned reflexes, Pavlov holds, follows an inhibition of a conditioned reflex, when the inhibition spreads over the entire cortex. In this dog drowsiness and sleep came first, and the cessation of the salivary flow followed, most probably because the action of the conditioned stimulus could not be exerted on the sleeping animal. (Kleitman concluded) that there was no inhibition of the conditioned reflex as such preceding the onset of sleep was indicated by the immediate resumption of the salivary flow when the animal was awakened." (p 218-219) (Kleitman 1930).

Kleitman and Camille (1932) undertook new research on decorticated dogs to quantify their sleep-waking cycle, since previous results from the literature, particularly Golz's (1892) finding, only stated that such animals are able to sleep. In these experiments, to keep the dogs alive, the ablation had to be performed in two steps, under barbital or ether anesthesia.

"Four dogs lived long enough after the second operation to permit satisfactory studies. Dog A lived for 158 days, B was killed one year after decortication, and C and D lived only for 17 and 14 days respectively. Each of the latter dogs, however, made a very quick recovery after the second operation -- C walking well the next day -- and was studied intensively, when he suddenly took a turn for the worse and died... Once asleep the dogs did not wake up spontaneously for periods of time varying from 30 minutes to several hours, but most frequently they slept from one to two hours. In the waking state they generally walked about, sometimes incessantly, sometimes with short periods of rest, for a long time ... As a rule, the walking was in a circle (Figure 7) ... On the average, the dogs spent from 10 to 45 minutes out of every hour in activity ... A slightly greater proportion of the time was spent in activity during the day than at night, but this was probably due to the disturbing noises of the laboratory during the working hours. The longest period of activity on record was 6 hours and 40 minutes of incessant walking. As a rule there were five or six periods of activity alternating with periods of rest and sleep each 24 hours." (p 476-477) ...

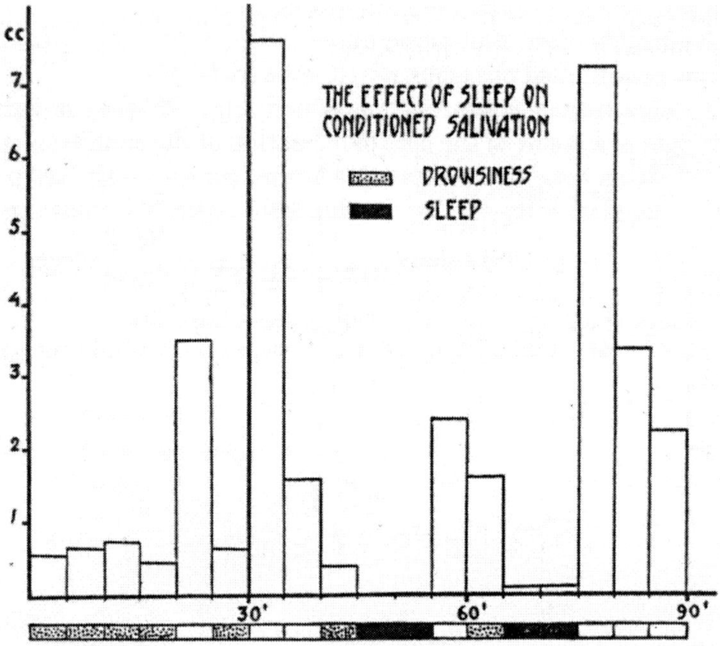

Figure 6. "A typical experiment showing the effect of drowsiness and sleep on the rate of salivary secretion of a dog, over successive 5 minute periods, before and after injection of morphine. During the first 20 minutes the dog was drowsy (eyes semi-closed) and the secretion rate was 0.4 to 0.7 cc over five minutes. During the next five minutes the dog was kept awake and the quantity of saliva rose to 3.5 cc. Permitted to become drowsy again, the dog secreted only 0.6 cc. in the last five minutes before the injection. After the injection of morphine the dog secreted 7.6 cc. and 1.6 cc. over the first two five-minute periods, respectively. She then became very drowsy, and the 0.4 cc. shown for the third period was actually collected in the first two minutes of that period. During the fourth and fifth periods the dog was definitively asleep and snoring, with no saliva coming out of the fistula for 13 minutes. The dog was then awakened and kept awake for the sixth period, during which she secreted 2.4 cc. Somewhat drowsy again during the seventh period, the secretion fell to 1.6 cc., and the dog was asleep during the eighth and ninth periods, when only 1.1 cc. was collected for each of the periods. Aroused again and kept awake, the secretion of saliva over the next three periods was 7.2 cc., 3.3 cc. and 2.2 cc. respectively" (P 218). Reprinted from *American Journal of Physiology*.

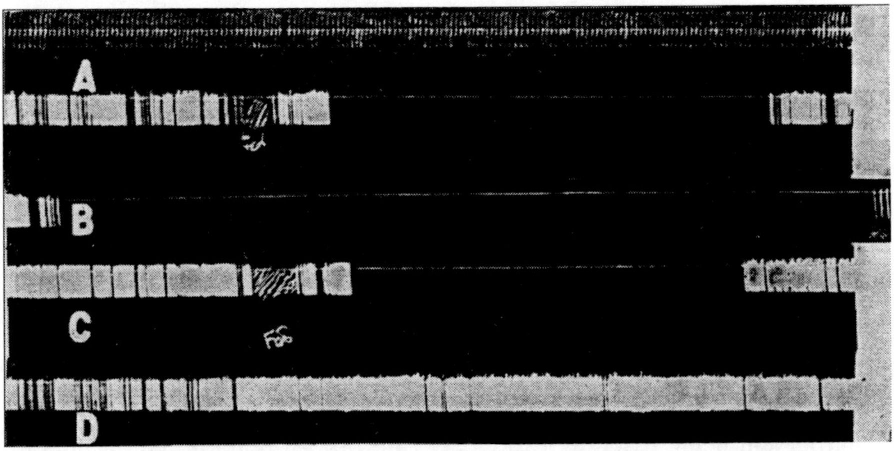

Figure 7. "A signal magnet records the activity of decorticated dog A, with each mark on the paper representing, as a rule, one circular walking movement. When the dog runs the marks coalesce, forming a band. Time in minutes, total time of each record about three hours. Recordings A and C show the short lasting activity after feeding (indicated by oblique marks), followed by about one and a half hours of rest. Recording B shows a rest period of three hours' duration, and recording D, a period of activity lasting more than three hours" (p 477). Reprinted from *American Journal of Physiology*.

> ... We see that the diurnal sleep, developed around the 24-hour cycle of day and night, is thus a definitely cortical phenomenon, has its center or is localized in the cerebral cortex, disappears when the cortex is removed ... That the subcortical sleep tendencies are ever ready to exert their action (the two authors mentioned first Mauthner's (1890) results) is demonstrated by the fact that most people can fall asleep not only at their habitual bedtime, but almost at any time, if a condition is brought about where the number of afferent impulses reaching the cerebral cortex is greatly reduced ..."
>
> ... There is no conflict between the subcortical and the cortical theories of sleep. The first account for sleep in general, the second for the special diurnal type of sleep seen only in higher animals and in man." (p 480) (Kleitman and Camille 1932).

Concerning Kleitman's general assertions (1927, 1932) that sleep occurs through a 'decrease in the number of afferent impulses' and 'fatigue of the neuromuscular mechanism', which was the only accepted theory in those days (referred to as 'deafferentation') (see Moruzzi, 1964), it can be argued that Kleitman's with his last paper probably submitted in 1931 could not be aware of the result of Hess (1931) showing that sleep can be induced by diencephalic stimulation; those results suggested that there was an active, and not only passive, process at the origin of sleep (see the beautiful discussion of the ins and outs of Hess's results by Jouvet (1972).

The same year, Kleitman (1932) again working alone, developed two new methods to measure human behavior in bed. He wanted to quantify the duration and amplitude of movements during the night. "Although it has been shown repeatedly that one stirs and turns over several times per hour during sleep, it has never been determined how much time one spends in these movements, or by difference what part of the time given to sleep one really lies still." (p 390). As we are essentially concerned by the results of such research, it does not seem worthwhile to describe in detail here his first new method, involving the opening and closing of an electrical circuit, with the quantification being made by two clocks, the first working at the opening of and the second at the closing of the movements. What is more important is to show the obtained results. "The sleep of three persons has been studied. The time spent in movement was very small, varying somewhat in the different subjects, and in the same subject during different nights. Subject C. spent from 34" to 87" and an average of 57" per hour in movement during sleep (based on 12 nights); subject M. from 13" to 28" and an average of 21" (11 nights); subject K. from 28" to 79" and an average of 49 (16 nights)... Thus, even though one moves very often, one still lies immovably about 59 minutes out of every hour." (p 390-391). Then, measuring the displacement in the bed during night: "The sum-total of the displacements … in subject C. varied from 72.8 to 139.5 cm. (6 nights); subject M. from 43.7 to 97.0 cm (6 nights)" (p 391). The nature of the device involved that these latter results should be doubled to obtain the true value. Kleitman indicated that his two devices are easy to be used at home. Interestingly, he mentioned the assistance in the research of N.R. Cooperman, and F.J. Mullin, who subsequently published several papers with him. Today, this kind of movement quantification generally involves wrist recording devices (Kripke, 1978).

Kleitman (1933) studied diurnal variations in intellectual and other types of cognitive performance.

> "To avoid the disturbing effects of the presence of an observer it was decided to use only such tests as could be performed on the subject by himself. To make these tests as soon as one woke up in the morning and just before going to bed, they had to be done in the subject home and therefore without any special apparatus. Of the six subjects used, two slept in the laboratory and they performed tasks requiring recording and other apparatus." (p 451).

There were six tasks (two with cards, mirror-image drawing, copying syllables, transcription of letters into a code, multiplication of eight-digit numbers). In the laboratory, the subjects had to hold a metal stylus in holes of different diameters, and their ability to stand upright with their eyes closed was also tested. The author provided a table (Table 6) with detailed numerical results.

Table 6. Performance and body temperature in humans

TYPE OF TEST	NUMBER OF SUBJECTS	NUMBER OF DAYS	7 A.M.	8 A.M.	12 M.	6 P.M.	11 P.M.
Dealing 156 playing cards	1	29	50.1	48.2	47.1	47.4	49.8
Sorting 156 playing cards	3	69	135	129	125	127	133
Mirror drawing of star	3	69	38.4	37.5	35.3	36.3	37.6
Code transcription, 400 letters	4	64	407	362	344	350	364
Copying text of 400 letters	3	56	291	267	256	259	266
Multiplication of 8 digit number by 8 digit number	3	69	427	409	371	373	384
Body temperature (mouth)	5	108	97.64	97.71	98.21	98.33	97.73

The average time, in seconds, required to perform certain tests and the average body temperature, in degrees Fahrenheit, at different hours of the day. Reprinted from *American Journal of Physiology*.

Conclusion: "There is a diurnal variation in the speed and accuracy of performance in Man, with a maximum in the afternoon and minima early in the morning and late at night (p 456) ... This parallelism was seen also in the test of readiness ... and in swaying of the body." (p 453) Kleitman (1933).

In 1933 also, Kleitman and Doktorsky (1933) studied the variation of temperature in relation to motor activity and sleep in humans.

> "It is well-known that the temperature of homeothermal animals is really not constant, but shows fluctuations of one or more degrees under different conditions. Muscular activity produces a temporary rise in body temperature which may be subjectively felt. The most regular change in temperature is associated with the twenty-four hour period of day and night, most individuals showing a well-marked diurnal temperature curve with a maximum in the afternoon and a minimal in the early hours of the morning. The fact that one's temperature begins to fall long before bedtime and follows its usual curve if one stays up all the night has been considered as showing that sleep is not directly responsible for the night temperature ...

... We reinvestigated the effect of position of the body and of sleep upon rectal temperature by the use of an electrical resistance recording thermometer which permits us to read the temperature with an accuracy of 0.02° Fahrenheit." (p 340).

Heart rate, respiration and (sometimes) blood pressure were measured in most cases.

While the authors provided a table with quantitative results of temperature variations for four subjects during different waking states and sleep. Figure 8 provides a clear enough view of the evolution of the temperature.

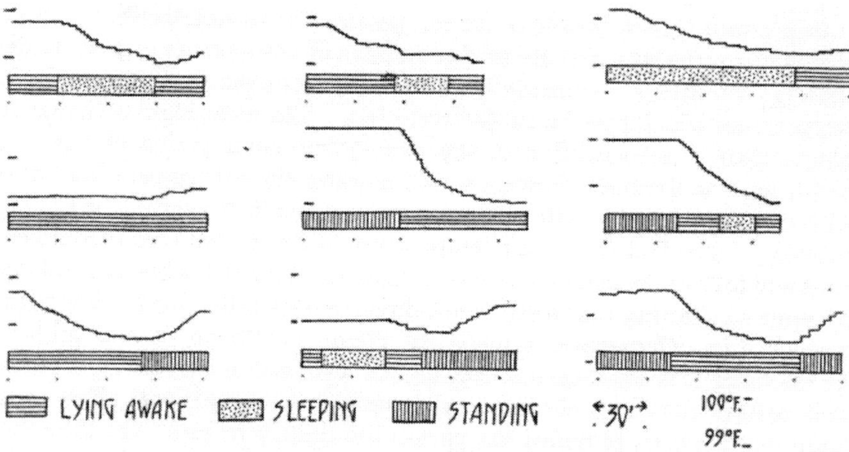

Figure 8. The effect of lying awake, sleeping and standing on rectal temperature in Man. Reprinted from *American Journal of Physiology*.

"It may be concluded that a change in the position of the body from vertical to horizontal leads to a fall in temperature ... Under ordinary conditions, going to bed at night when the muscle tonus is low, leads to a further decrease in tonus -- as indicated by the low temperature --, thus producing an additional decrease in the number of proprioceptive impulses reaching the cerebral cortex and making continued wakefulness impossible. After the onset of sleep the temperature may or may not show a renewed drop, depending upon the degree of muscular relaxation already attained, and upon the time of the day or night. For the same reason awakening may result in a rise, no change, or in a fall in temperature." (p 343) (Kleitman and Doktorsky 1933).

Kleitman's next 1933 paper was devoted to the study of motility and temperature during sleep (Kleitman et al., 1933), as all three were the primary scientists involved in the measurements performed on the eight subjects participating in the experiment.

> "We decided to determine as closely as possible the actual time spent in stirring during sleep. We also wanted to record the temperature of the sleeper in order to detect a possible connection between motility and the temperature level or temperature changes during sleep." (p 574).

The authors first showed, in a detailed figure, a device for simultaneously recording movements and rectal temperature; this was an extension of a previously described method (Kleitman, 1932). The quantitative results are shown in Table 7.

Table 7. Motility during sleep

SUBJECT	NUMBER OF NIGHTS	NUMBER OF MOVEMENTS			PERCENTAGE FALLING IN SECOND HALF OF NIGHT		
		Major	Minor	Total	Major	Minor	Total
B. O. B.	6	14.2	25.2	39.4	71	63	66
N. B.	6	16.4	18.7	35.1	65	65	65
E. B.	5	20.8	34.1	54.9	66	69	68
N. R. C.	86	27.5	19.5	47.0	58	55	57
A. I. D.	5	11.0	11.5	22.5	62	69	66
N. K.	11	22.6	13.5	36 1	61	59	60
F. J. M.	66	12.8	28.3	41.1	66	63	64
S. P.	5	16.4	23.3	39.7	67	60	63

The average number of movements during the night and the percentage occurring during the second half of the night. Reprinted from *American Journal of Physiology*.

> "The time actually spent in motility was much smaller than expected on the basis of the frequency with which movements occurred during the night. In extensive series of observations on three subjects the time taken from rest by movements of all kinds, for each hour of staying in bed, was found to be on the average, 43.0 seconds (K., 38 nights), 34.1 seconds (C., 66 nights), and 19.7 seconds (M., 59 nights). From two to four minutes was all that was not spent in complete immobility during the usual night's sleep ... For the above-mentioned three subjects the average hourly displacements were 15.4, 14.0 and 7.4 cm. corresponding to hourly mobility of 43.0, 34.1 and 19.7 seconds (p 578-579) ... The greater number of longer periods of immobility fell in the first half of the night» (p 579) ... During the night sleep our subjects executed, on the average from 11 to 28 major movements, probably involving a change in the

position of the sleeper, and the average total number of movements varied from 20 to 55" (p 583) …

"... The temperature changes are of interest mainly because they were recorded synchronously with motility during sleep ... The most characteristic drop in temperature occurred shortly after going to bed and was undoubtedly due to the assumption of the horizontal position (as shown previously by the same team (Kleitman et al., 1933) ... (However, contrary to daytime waking) there is no definite connection between motility and temperature changes ... and considerable motility may take place without a change in temperature, and vice-versa." (p 582) (Figure 9).

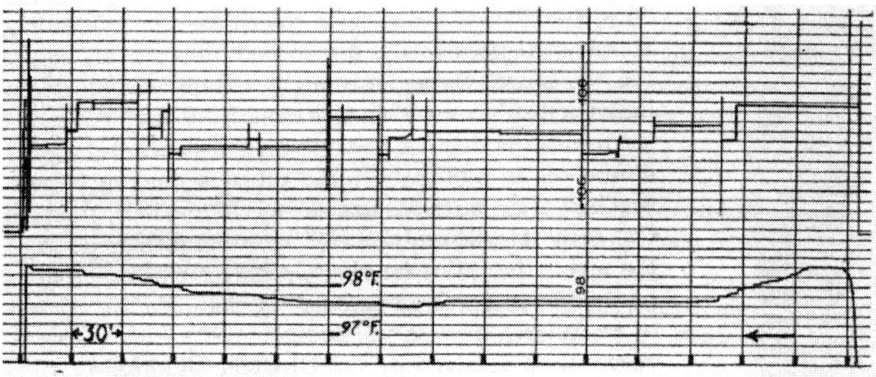

Figure 9. Reduced reproduction of an actual recording of motility (above) and rectal temperature (below) performed on subject Mullin. The signal magnet recording has been omitted. Time scale: 30 minutes. Reprinted from *American Journal of Physiology*.

… "There is a suggestion that a higher temperature (during sleep) may mean a greater inclination to spontaneous awakening and ability of being aroused by outside stimulation." (p 584).

Finally,

"The observations scattered over more than a year were grouped under two headings: summer-autumn (May 17- Nov. 16) and winter-spring (Nov. 17- May 16), but most of the data were accumulated in the autumn and in the winter ... It is evident that temperature level and motility are higher in the autumn than in the winter." (p 583) (Kleitman et al., 1933).

The fact that the temperature decrease was more pronounced in the first half of night can be interpretated as occurring in deep slow wave sleep (SWS), stages III and IV.

Finally, Kleitman (Mullin et al. 1933), reported on the effects of alcohol and caffeine on motility and temperature during sleep. As done previously, indeed in every one of Kleitman's papers, an attentive study of the literature was first performed. Because the previously available results provided no precise indications about administered doses, Kleitman and his colleagues reinvestigated the problem using the same recording method as in their previous research (Kleitman and Doktorsky, 1933). "This enabled us to measure the total time spent in movement, as well as the distribution of that time. We also recorded the total centimeter displacement of the bed-spring, and the frequency and amplitude of individual movements. In some cases we took continuous rectal temperature records throughout the night ... 60 to 75 cc of 95 per cent alcohol diluted to a 19 per cent concentration were taken forty-five minutes to one hour before retiring ... The coffee drinks were brewed from varying amounts of ground coffee bean (25 to 75 grams) using three 5-ounce cups of water, percolated for seven minutes. One cup of coffee was taken at each three consecutive forty-five minute intervals before going to bed ... (In each case there was a control experiment). Eight male subjects were employed in this study. The most extensive observations were made on ourselves." (p 479-480). Among the subjective feelings, Kleitman's own can be mentioned: "N. K. an abstainer from coffee, complained of a 'miserable night' after the consumption of three cups of the beverage made from a total of twenty-five grams of ground coffee beans." (!) (p 479-480). The quantitative results are summarized in (Figure 10).

> … "Alcohol decreased both the major and minor movements occurring during the first part of the night, the effect being particularly striking in the two first hours, and increased in the last half of the night (p 482-483) ... In the case of caffeine, the large doses gave a great increase in the number of movements occurring during the first half of the night, often because the inability of the subject to go to sleep … Alcohol always caused a lowered temperature during the first half of the night and an increased temperature during the second half." (p 484). An observation made during waking while sitting showed a similar drop. "The large doses of caffeine always gave a significantly higher temperature at corresponding times during the night's sleep." (p 484) (Mullin et al. 1933).

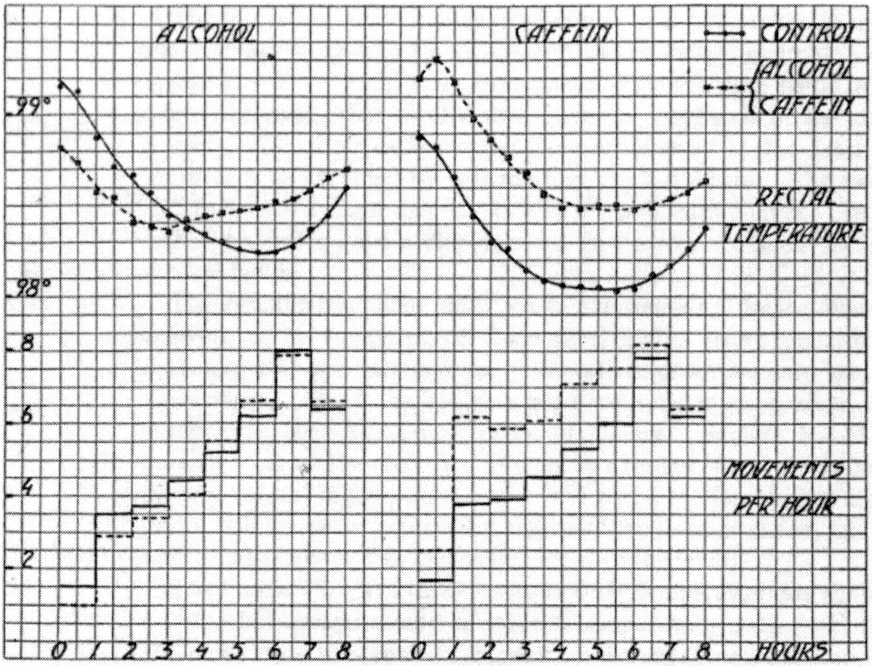

Figure 10. The effect of alcohol (300 and 375 cc doses of 19 per cent alcohol) and caffeine (4 and 6 beans) on body temperature and motility of the first author of this paper. Reprinted from *American Journal of Physiology*.

To conclude, the authors, without being able to provide any definite explanations at the time, stated that there was a causal relationship between the lowering of temperature by alcohol during the first half of the night, its rise during the second part, and motility, which is affected in exactly the same manner. In the same way, they had no definite explanations for the increase in body temperature that occurs during the second half of the night following alcohol consumption.

In 1934, Kleitman's group (Cooperman et al., 1934) performed a new study on the subjective and objective consequences of prolonged sleep deprivation. A total of 13 periods of 60 hours each were studied, using similar tests as in their previous research devoted to deprivation (Lee and Kleitman, 1923). The additional tasks concerned hand steadiness, visual acuity and the threshold of cutaneous sensitivity to touch and pain. Six male subjects underwent one or more sleepless periods.

"Subjectively, it was easily ascertained that it was much more difficult to keep awake, as well as to perform the various tasks of the tests between 3 and 6.00 a.m. than later in the following day ... The subject's performance was influenced not only by the time of day or night, but also by what he has been doing during the half-hour or so preceding the test. Some of the subjects became hyper-irritable and reacted in an uncalled-for manner at the slightest provocation ... Frequently their behavior resembled that of persons who were under the influence of an intoxicating dose of alcohol ...

... Objectively ... we found no significant changes in reaction time or the ability to name 100 colors, but marked changes in the ability to stand upright with one's eyes closed. In recording the time required to name successive 100 colored squares in a 400-colored test, we observed a slowing up in the naming of the third and fourth hundreds only...

... As regards the new tests, visual acuity did not show any consistent deviation from the normal, but there was a decrease in hand steadiness on the third day of the period of wakefulness ... While the threshold for touch sensibility remained practically unchanged, the threshold for pain sensitivity was greatly reduced in every one of the six subjects, on every abstention from sleep...

... The sleep following a period of wakefulness of 60 hours was characterized by a considerable increase in duration ... it amounted, on the average, to twelve hours ..., a marked decrease in motility, both as regards frequency, extent, and duration of movement." (p 591-592) (Cooperman et al., 1934) (Figure 11).

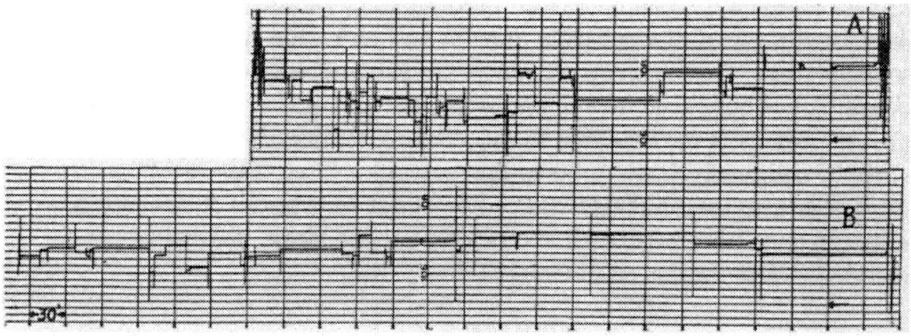

Figure 11. Typical recording of motility during sleep in a subject. A. Control night's sleep over eight hours' duration. B. A longer night's sleep following a period of wakefulness of 62 hours. Reprinted from *American Journal of Physiology.*

A short abstract on reaction time in relation to body temperature was published in 1935 (Kleitman et al., 1935). The best is to include it here in its entirety. "Simple reaction time to light and sound, and reaction time with choice to colored lights were studied on five male subjects. The reaction time in all cases was high early in the day, decreased to a minimum during the afternoon and rose during the evening. Simultaneous determinations of the mouth temperature revealed an inverse relationship between changes in body temperature and reaction time, particularly reaction time with choice. The lighter the temperature the quicker the response. The speed of response followed pretty closely the diurnal curve of body temperature, in the same manner as did previously reported diurnal variations in performance and in steadiness (see Kleitman and Doktorsky, 1933)".

The next paper was published in 1937. It concerned the establishment of the diurnal temperature cycle (Kleitman et al., 1937).

> "Since the diurnal alternation of sleep and wakefulness is absent at birth, one would expect to find no diurnal variation in body temperature in the young infant. However, data available in the literature show that even the new-born exhibit such a daily variation in temperature, sometimes amounting to over one-half a degree Centigrade." (p 48).

In the following paragraph, the authors analyzed the known data in the literature. It is noteworthy that for the first time, the authors quantified the results in degrees centigrade.

> "Our own observations were made on new-born babies at the Chicago Lying-In Hospital and on older babies and children at the Bobs Robert Memorial Hospital. The new-borns were entirely normal, and the older ones were in hospital for observation or for correction of nutritional disorders, and with some few exceptions, were not 'sick' and did not have fever. Their rectal temperature was determined every two hours, except between midnight and 8 a.m. Only one reading was made at 4.00 a.m ... The immediate environmental temperature was read off a thermometer attached to the child's bed. The periods of sleep and wakefulness, of eating, and of activity were also noted." (p 49).

Table 8 shows the results for the different ages.

> "Our results demonstrate that while there may be a diurnal fluctuation in body temperature even in young infants, the diurnal temperature cycle, in the sense of a regularly recurring and superimposable variation, first appears during the second year of the child's life... The factors responsible are partly exogenous and partly endogenous. Among the former, the diurnal variation in environmental temperature is of minor, if any importance; the feeding routine which

early in life is confined to the waking hours of the mother is probably of greater influence ... The endogenous factor is probably the development of the nervous system which permits an adaptation of wakefulness and sleep to the alternating cycle of day and night. In passing from the polyphasic type of existence characteristic of the new-born to the monophasic seen in older children and adults, one of the first learned performances is sleeping through the whole night by skipping one feeding, and the gradual lengthening of the daytime periods of wakefulness. Instead of sleep being the prevalent mode of existence, with wakefulness interrupting it periodically for short intervals of time, we end up with the waking state comprising 15 to 17 hours out of the 24, and one continuous period of sleep, usually during the hours of darkness ... Another important feature … is the daytime temperature plateau with a rather sharp drop in the evening and an equally sharp rise in the early hours of the morning ... The body temperature begins to drop in the evening long before the onset of sleep, and likewise begins to rise sharply shortly after midnight, or long before awakening. If the sharp evening temperature fall is indicative of marked muscular relaxation, it would mean that the relaxation is the cause rather than the effect of sleep, and that it plays an important part in the mechanism of the diurnal cycle." (p 52-53) (Kleitman et al., 1937).

Table 8. Diurnal variation of temperature during infant growth

AGE GROUP	NUMBER OF SUBJECTS	VARIATION IN INDIVIDUAL DIURNAL TEMPERATURE RANGES	GROUP AVERAGE OF THE DIURNAL TEMPERATURE RANGE (AR)	THE AVERAGE DIURNAL TEMPERATURE CURVE FOR THE AGE GROUP			AR/RA
				High	Low	Range (RA)	
		°C.		°C.	°C.	°C.	
New-born	10	0.35–0.74	0.62	36.95	36.68	0.27	2.30
1–5 mo.	5	0.62–1.02	0.80	37.28	36.72	0.56	1.43
7–11 mo.	6	0.74–1.15	0.98	37.38	36.56	0.82	1.20
14–22 mo.	6	1.18–1.80	1.67	37.51	35.95	1.56	1.07
3–6 yr.	4	1.39–1.86	1.56	37.50	36.15	1.35	1.16
7–13 yr.	4	1.10–1.82	1.44	37.73	36.36	1.37	1.05

'The ratio of the average diurnal temperature range in a given age group (AR) to the range of the average, or composite, diurnal body temperature curve for that group (RA)". Reprinted from *American Journal of Physiology*.

The second paper from 1937 was devoted to the threshold needed for awakening by auditory stimulation (Mullin et al., 1937). The results of this experiment were obtained on five dogs and six men.

One hundred and sixty-three measurements were performed on dogs from the onset of sleep (Figure 12).

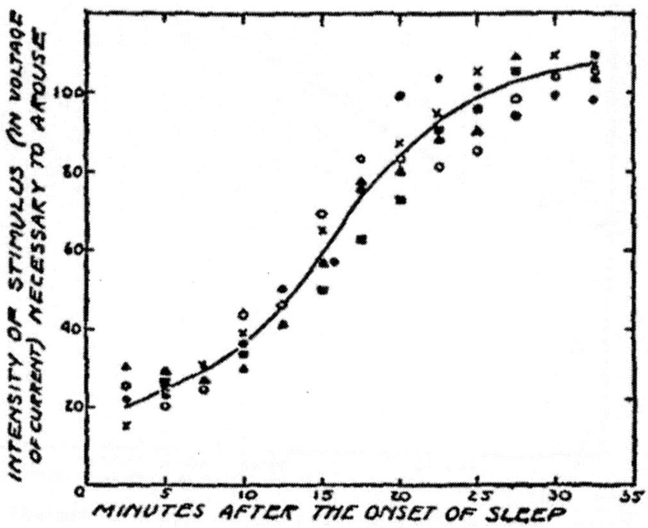

Figure 12. Average arousal threshold obtained from five dogs. Reprinted from *Journal of Experimental Psychology*.

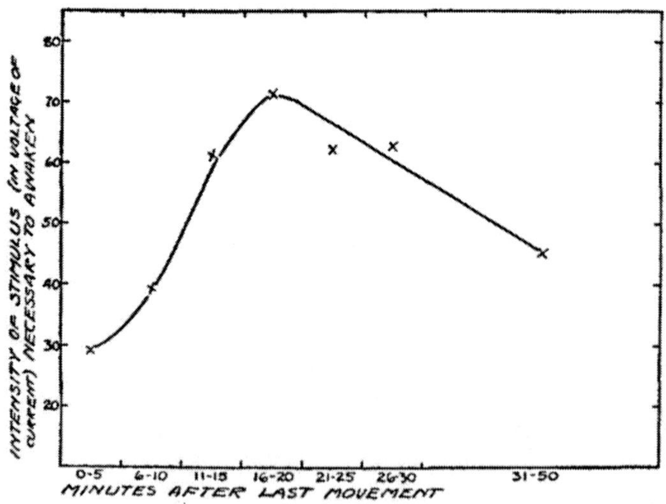

Figure 13. Average arousal threshold obtained in men. The results are the mean of a total of three hundred and twenty-five observations. Reprinted from *Journal of Experimental Psychology*.

In the six male subjects that were also studied, the intensities needed to awaken the subjects were quantified from the occurrence of the last movement after sleep onset. According to the authors, the curve was globally the same as in dogs (Figure 13).

> "With a few exceptions, the longer the interval of quiescence between pairs of successive movements the higher the intensity of stimulus necessary to awaken, and the more prolonged is the decrease in irritability, no matter what time of night this occurred." (p 92).

The authors also presented results showing the evolution of the arousal threshold during the night (Figure 14).

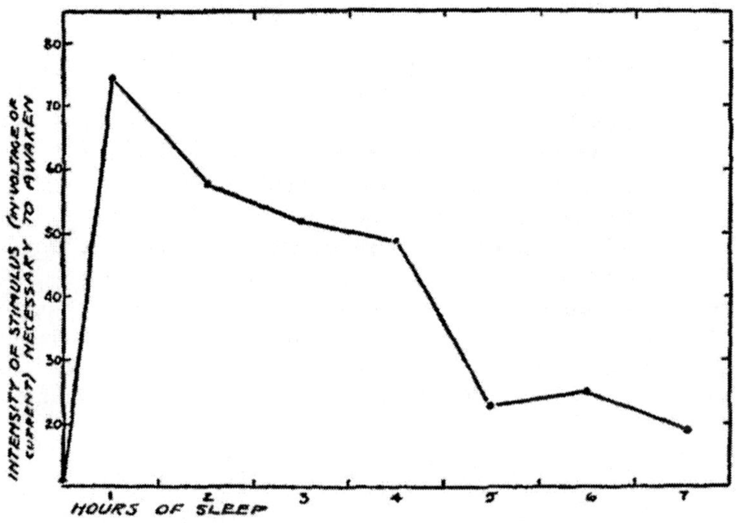

Figure 14. Mean value of arousal threshold during subjects' night sleep. Reprinted from *Journal of Experimental Psychology*.

Following up on his previous study (Kleitman, 1933) which had revealed a relationship between performance and body temperature, in 1938 Kleitman et al., (1938) reported further studies on this relationship. It followed a short, previously published abstract (Kleitman et al., 1935).

> "The performances selected for this purpose were purely sensory-motor: reaction to light and reaction to sound, and sensory-mental-motor: choice reactions to light and sound... Five male graduate students and an instructor participated, each acting alternatively as subject and observer."

(p 495). “The subjects were tested in mean from 9 a.m. to 9 p.m. In one subject up to 11 p.m. The complete test comprised: 1/ A simple reaction time to white light; 2/ A simple reaction time to sound of a telegraphic key; 3/ A choice reaction which was response to green light, but not red; 4/ Another choice reaction: response to sound of a bell, but not to the telegraphic key. Temperature was determined by a mouth clinical thermometer for five minutes after each test.” (p 495-496) ...

“... [A] fairly good relationship between body temperature and reaction time was observed regardless of the time of day, indicating that there is probably no diurnal reaction time curve independent of the temperature.” (p 497) (Figure 15).

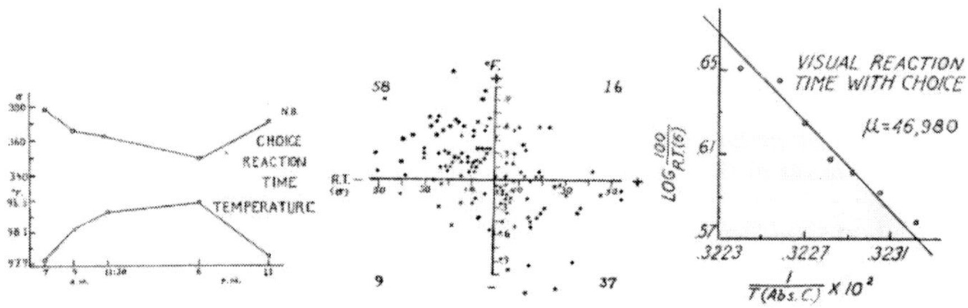

Figure 15. Simultaneous variations in performance and body temperature. " Left: Diurnal variation in reaction time to choice visual stimuli for one subject. Upper curve, reaction time in sigma. Lower curve, temperature in degrees Fahrenheit. Centre: The relationship between change in body temperature and change in visual reaction time in a subject, based upon 120 pairs of observations, usually separated by two or three hours. Body temperature changes are plotted along the x-axes and reaction time changes along the y-axes. In most cases, a change in body temperature in one direction is accompanied by a change in reaction time in the opposite direction: 95 cases show this relationship, compared to 25 cases where the body temperature and reaction time varied in the same direction. Right: The relationship between body temperature and reaction time to choice visual stimuli. The curve is fitted by the method of least squares” (p 499). Reprinted from *American Journal of Physiology*.

“There is a definite difference in the degree of mental activity required of the subject between the performance designated as simple reaction and that called reaction with choice. In the former alertness is all that is required, but in the latter where the individual is to respond to one type of signal and not to another, analysis and judgment are the added requirements. That is reflected in the longer time, roughly one-tenth of a second, needed for reaction with choice ... It is significant that the effect of temperature is more marked with respect to reaction time with choice than in simple reaction (p 500) ...

... Assuming that the effect of temperature indicates that we are dealing with a chemical phenomenon, there are two interpretations of the relationship between temperature and reaction time possible: either a, mental processes represent chemical reactions in themselves, or b, the speed of thinking depends upon the level of metabolic activity of the cells of the cerebral cortex, and by raising the latter through an increase in body temperature we indirectly speed up the thought processes." (p 501) (Kleitman et al., 1938).

Also in 1938, the group (Mullin and Kleitman 1938) quantified the arousal threshold involved in the response to auditory stimuli of increasing intensity lasting for 10 seconds. The subjects had to answer 'I hear it'. More than 1000 individual thresholds were studied in 20 sleepers: "eight normal adults, five normal children from 4 to 7 years of age and seven feeble-minded adults with I.Q. ratings of 30 to 50." (p 478). 'Going to sleep' was determined by the drop of a paper held in the hand. Complementary criteria were changes in respiration, muscle twitching, etc. Figure 16 summarizes the results obtained in the three samples of subjects.

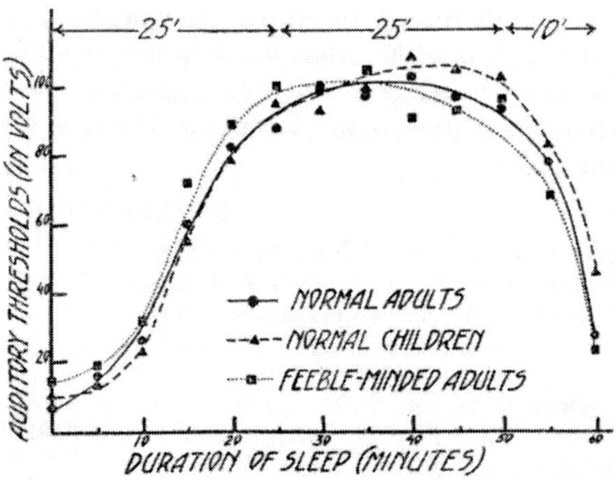

Figure 16. Superimposed curves of auditory arousal threshold during the first hour of sleep. There were 996 determinations made on eight normal adults, 571 on five children and 668 on seven feeble-minded subjects. Reprinted from *American Journal of Physiology*.

The results are nearly identical in the three groups. The highest arousal threshold was observed about 25 minutes after sleep onset, before a decrease to the waking level. The data confirmed those of a previous study performed on dogs, in which the assessment was stopped after 30 minutes, thus before dropping (curve in S), as well as those from a determination made at the very beginning of the night in humans (Mullin et al., 1937).

> "The fact that the curves for children, adults and the feeble-minded are so closely alike indicates that neither physical nor intellectual development modifies the process of the development of the state of sleep … Lastly, the failure of the curve to start de novo after the sleeper had responded to stimulation suggests that he was not totally awake at the time, and this is supported by his frequently not being able to recall whether he had responded or not. It suggests, furthermore, that it is not necessary for an individual to be fully awake in order to perform simple acts, and we undoubtedly go through a number of such semi-waking states during an ordinary night's sleep." (p 480) (Mullin and Kleitman 1938).

In his last paper published in 1939, before the publication in the same year of the first edition of *Sleep and Wakefulness* (1939), Kleitman published the results of research performed with, in alphabetic order, Blake, Gerard and Kleitman, (1939). This study represented the beginning of his work on brain electrophysiology in humans, which was later most often called EEG. This study also examined, or recalled from previous work (Berger, 1929), additional major properties of sleep as compared to waking.

This paper first provided a new classification of sleep-waking stages based on the different EEG activities. This system differed from previously proposed systems, particularly that introduced by Loomis et al. (1937) (Table 9).

Table 9. Sleep stage nomenclature

	Aomplitude Alpha	Amplitude Delta	Amplitude 14 per sec.	Depth of sleep	Present Nomenclature	Nomenclature of Loomis et al.
1	++	-	-	Awake	Alpha	A. Interrupted alpha B. Low voltage C. Spindles
2	+	++	+	Light sleep	Alpha+delta (+ 14 per sec.)	
3	-	+++	+	Deep sleep	Delta (+14 per sec.)	D. Spindles + random E. Random
4	-	-	+	Light sleep	Null (or low voltage)	B. Low voltage
5	(+)	-	(+)	Sleep to wake	Intermitent alpha	B. to A. Low voltage to interrupted alpha
6	+	-	-	Awake	Alpha (low intensity)	

Designation of author's sleep-waking stage nomenclature (center) based on EEG patterns, compared to the previous classification (right), for example as given by Loomis et al. (1937). It is of interest that the authors spoke about 14/sec activity instead of spindles, and of null activity for low amplitude (rapid) activity. Marks (+ and -) have been intensified. Reprinted from *Journal of Neurophysiology*.

Then, the authors gave a schema of the distribution of brain potentials observed at night (Figure 17).

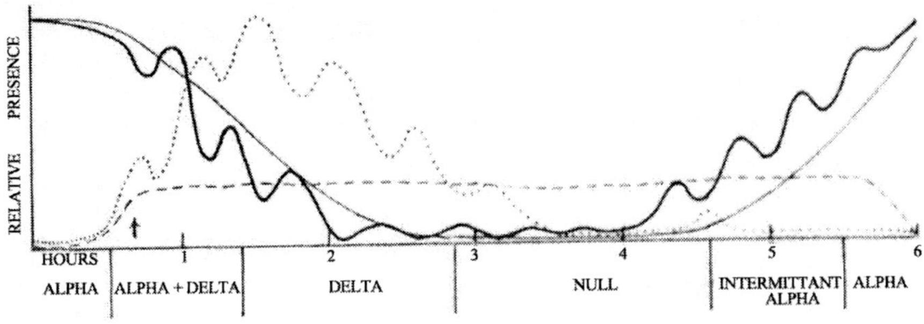

Figure 17. Co-variation of EEG activity and body temperature during the night. The heavy black line represents the level of alpha rhythm, the thin line the evolution of temperature, and the wavy lines the changes in waves due to shifting of the sleep state. The arrow indicates sleep onset. Reprinted from *Journal of Neurophysiology*.

The authors noted that the arousal thresholds roughly paralleled the delta activity curve. The lightening of sleep in the second part of the night, as shown by low voltage activity (null stage), heralded the longer morning REM sleep periods. Several examples of EEG activities are provided, but one is particularly interesting since it shows brain activity during dreaming, confirming Loomis et al.'s (1937) results (Fig 18).

> "In nine-tenths of the trials, when alpha waves had been missing for 9 sec. (and no delta waves were present) the subject could remember a dream." (p 53).

It is noteworthy that, as a result of the present findings, as confirmed by Lufkin (1968), when Kleitman later sent Aserinsky to go to learn eye movement recording in Jacobson's laboratory (Jacobson, 1930, 1938), he probably already anticipated the result he was later to obtain.

The movements recorded by the bed box, as well as the muscle potentials taken from the head leads, showed that: "movement is accompanied by a shift of potentials towards lighter sleep in nine-tenths of the present cases, by no change the remaining times." (p 59).

The study of body temperature showed that "a decline in muscle tone should decrease body temperature gradually; an increase in tone should raise temperature, but not so quickly as it restores the alpha rhythm. Both the alpha rhythm presence and the temperature are lower in the morning after waking than they were the previous evening." (p 55).

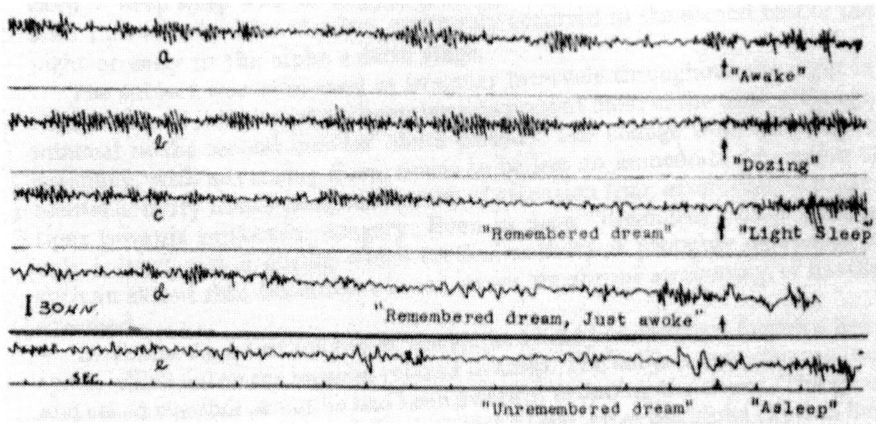

Figure 18. Occurrence of low voltage EEG activity during established sleep during which dreaming was reported twice. Reprinted from *Journal of Neurophysiology*.

The authors also performed 100-hour sleep deprivations by benzedrine taken at intervals. "Slow waves predominated with the subject recumbent, even though talking or with the eyes open, and they disappeared only when the he made an extreme effort to concentrate." (p 55). In the same way, eleven narcoleptic subjects showed less alpha activity when lying down and "delta waves at relatively higher levels of consciousness than in normal sleep." (p 59) (Blake, Gerard and Kleitman, 1939). Finally, benzedrine diminished delta waves, and alcohol enhanced them.

It must be mentioned that this research followed other results obtained by Blake and Gerard (1937), who had attentively studied EEG activities during sleep; these authors, along with others (Derbyshire et al. 1936, Loomis et al. 1937), observed a stage with "feeble irregular potentials", that was qualified as 'lighter sleep' (p 702), even though "the test sound evoked no response" (p 696), showing an increased arousal (or EEG change) threshold. Also, in cats, Klaue (1937) (also quoted by Kleitman 1939) had described a *Tiefer* Schlaf (deep sleep) with low amplitude cortical activity, "complete muscular relaxation … and numerous jerks of extremities" (p 514). These results announced (the later-confirmed) specific changes in the arousal threshold during sleep (Dement, 1958 ; Benoit and Bloch 1960 ; Jouvet et al., 1960) in cats, (Aserinsky and Kleitman 1953a ; Dement and Kleitman, 1957a; Williams et al., 1962) in humans. These first features already were strong indices of higher arousal threshold during REM sleep.

It is of interest that Kleitman, who was acknowledged at the end of the paper of Blake and Gerard for his 'constructive criticism of the work', was not a co-author, since the paper refers to an unpublished result of Mullin and Kleitman. It was possible that Kleitman had first wanted to confirm Blake and Gerard's (1937) results, which was ultimately done in Kleitman's final paper from 1939, discussed above. Following Hartmut Schulz's suggestion (March 2013), it is possible that Helen Blake being a graduate student in Gerard's laboratory in the Department of Physiology and having received her PhD in 1936, supervised by Gerard, this may explain the tandem authorship of the 1937 paper. Since Kleitman had his own laboratory in the same department, the interaction between the three persons may have been intensified thereafter, leading to the triple authorship of the 1939 paper.

The first paper to be published during the Second World War (Kleitman, 1943) was devoted to workers' schedules, which was particularly important at the time as there were many highly active factories manufacturing armaments without interruption.

> "When a night-worker complains of his inability to sleep well in the daytime, he unintentionally conveys the information that he is very sleepy at night, when he should be wide-awake at his bench or machine … The sleepiness of the unhappy night worker is not only due to his working during the customary hours of sleep, but also to the fact that he slept poorly the day before … Under ordinary routine conditions of existence, the peak or plateau of the temperature curve is reached some time during the afternoon, usually between 1 and 7 p.m. At that time our efficiency is greatest. The minimal body temperature is reached during the early morning hours, somewhere between 2 and 5 a.m. If one stays awake overnight, those are the hours of worst inefficiency and greatest difficulty of remaining awake … and drop in performance between 2 and 5 a.m. …
>
> … The application of these facts to the solution of the multiple shift problem has two aspects: (1) rotation or maintenance of shifts and (2) shift distribution or timing."

With respect to (1) the author discussed the advantages and disadvantages of rotations and maintenance of the shifts. Indeed, "it takes several weeks for a new 24-hour sleep-work-meals-leisure cycle to be properly established. Such achievement is wholly impossible under the system which prevails in some establishments of weekly or bi-weekly shift rotation, because the individual is not given a chance to adapt himself to a new routine… The way to overcome this effect is to keep each worker on a given shift for extended periods of time.” Concerning point 2, several kinds of shifts are proposed by Kleitman. The main proposal is the 3x8 hour shifts which are still the most frequently used today, and which he proposed as the best schedule to disturb at minima the workers, stating that this "shift timing has a number of advantages." (p 16) (Figure 19).

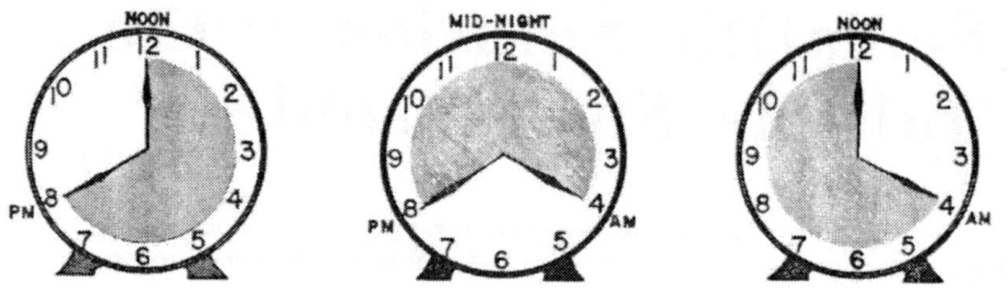

RED (Sunset) shift. Working hours from noon to 8 p.m. Evening and early night free for leisure activies. Sleep from 1 or 2 to 9 or 10 a.m.

WHITE (Victory) shift. Working hours from 8 p.m. to 4 a.m. Sleep from 5 a.m. to 1 p.m. Afternoon and early evening free for leisure

BLUE (Dawn) shift. Working hours from 4 a.m. to noon. Leisure in the afternoon. Sleeping from about 7 p.m. to 3 a.m.

Figure 19. Working schedules. Timing of rotation. On the left, the ‘RED (Sunset)’ shift Working hours from noon to 8 p.m. Evening and early night free for leisure activities. Sleep from 1 or 2 to 9 or 10 a.m. Centre. ‘White (Victory)’ shift. Working hours from 8 p.m. to 4 a.m. Sleep from about 5 a.m. to 1 p.m. Afternoon and early evening free for leisure. Right. ‘Blue (Dawn)’ shift. Working hours from 4 a.m. to noon. Leisure in the afternoon. Sleeping from about 7 p.m. to 3 a.m. Reprinted from *Mining Congress Journal.*

However, “with five eight-hour working shifts per week, the weekly holiday of two days may have an upsetting effect on the establishment and maintenance of this displacement cycle … One answer … is to decrease the weekend break to one day … Another solution … is to have the workers continue without interruptions on a seven-day per week basis for a number of weeks and then be given one week’s vacation.” (p 16). Two other suggestions were also provided: the 4x6-hour shift and the 10-hour shift for factories that were required to stop production for a number of hours each day. It would be interesting to have more information about the working conditions in those days to be able to better evaluate the novelty of Kleitman’s proposals.

In 1945, Kleitman published a paper in Science entitled, “The effect of motion pictures on body temperature.” (Kleitman 1945). This paper did not concern sleep but shows the breadth of his interests. Similarly, on a different non-sleep topic, Kleitman and Ramsaroop (1946) published a short communication on "Body temperature and cutaneous sensitivity to tingling and pain."

In 1947, with T. Engelman (by invitation), Kleitman published a short communication on the diurnal cycle of activity and body temperature in rabbits (Kleitman and Engelman, 1947). This work indirectly concerned rest and sleep. With free access to food, the activity of the animals was lower during the daytime, with a minimal level at noon, and highest during the night. Rectal temperatures were also lowest during the daytime but tended to rise during the evening. "When food was available only from 9-10 a.m. to 3-4 p.m., the animals quickly adapted themselves to this routine … Activity became more decidedly monophasic, increasing sharply in the morning … and continuing at high level during the day. The rectal temperature showed a marked rise during the feeding period, reaching its high level in the afternoon, instead of late in the evening." (p 143).

The next year, Kleitman et al., (1948) published a short communication on variations in human temperature, measuring the feet, toes, soles, and legs as well as the fingers, palms and forearms during waking and upon falling asleep. "The sudden steep rise in the temperature of the feet one or two hours before (sometimes immediately before or after) the onset of sleep has been interpreted as evidence of peripheral vasodilation due to a decrease in sympathetic activity, manifesting a 'vegetative preparedness for sleep' … In the pre-sleep hours of the evening, there is … a combination of two toe skin-temperature raising influences: meal and muscular relaxation. It therefore seems that the feet, especially the toes, exhibit vasomotor changes that are not characteristic of the skin as a whole, not even of the skin of the extremities, and changes in foot temperatures cannot be looked upon as variations in general sympathetic activity." (p 66).

The same year, Kleitman and Ramsaroop (1948) studied the periodicity of body temperature and heart rate. "It has been known for over a century that the human body temperature is not constant, but exhibits regularly recurring fluctuations. A diurnal, or 24-hour, cycle is related to the influence of the daily routine of work, meals, rest, and sleep." (p 1). This extensive paper, devoted to longer rhythm variations, came after an earlier paper studying temperature variations linked to ovulation (Kleitman, 1944). In this earlier paper, sleep was almost not taken into account at all, although the paper did note that workers adapted better to shifts of 3 to 4 hours when in the new schedule the onset of sleep was 3 hours later than usual, after 2 a.m. Temperature and heart rate variations were also extensively studied during the menstrual cycle and during pregnancy.

In 1949, Kleitman (1949a) published a very interesting short review on the sleep habits of children.

> "The child is born with certain capacities for learning, including the ability to synchronize, with ease or difficulty, the primitive sleep-wakefulness cycle with diurnal periodicity in his physical and social environment. To establish good sleep habits in children it is necessary to cooperate with the natural tendency to develop a persistent 24-hour rhythm, reinforcing the latter by the customary methods of conditioning." (p 66).
>
> "Many sleep disturbances in children cannot be foreseen and therefore have to be treated after they develop. Some are the result of poor sleep habits and can be overcome by replacing poor habits with good ones. Still better, such disturbances can be prevented by proper mental hygiene measures inaugurated as early in life as possible (p 63) … (For) going to bed in the evening … when the diurnal body temperature curve is fully established, physiological readiness for sleep (Schlafbereitschaft) is coupled with a rather sharp drop in temperature at a particular hour, making further maintenance of the waking state difficult or impossible. A definite familiar ritual of preparing for going to bed (washing, brushing teeth, changing into night clothes etc.) becomes a powerful suggestive influence in making the child psychologically, as well as physiologically, ready for sleep. Finally, friendly reassuring words from a parent, nurse, or older sibling, recitation of prayer, being covered and 'tucked in' for the night, can all be used to reinforce the time-conditioned onset of sleep." (p 64). Various rules regarding conditions for getting up in the morning, daytime naps, and duration of sleep, which are well known today, are also taken into account. In this latter paragraph the author distinguished 'morning persons' from 'evening persons' (see below). "Such extreme tendencies sometimes manifest themselves in children. Gentle efforts to shift the hours of onset and termination of sleep suffice, as a rule, to rectify a diurnal routine that is too much out of line with that of the rest of the family … The refractory child may be a future evening person." (p 65-66) (Kleitman 1949a).

Finally, this paper refers to the review discussed next as being in press.

Thus, also in 1949, Kleitman (1949b) wrote a major review devoted to biological rhythms and cycles. "This review of reviews though by no means exhaustive" (p 2) was very rich, and was devoted to rhythms that are shorter, equal or longer than 24 hours as observed in invertebrates and vertebrates, including mammals and Man. Recalling his own results on daily temperature variations, partly obtained in a cave with a stabilized temperature, he distinguished between the "so-called morning types (who) reach their maximum temperature early in the day," and whose performance "is better immediately upon getting up...", from the "evening type, who 'comes to life' toward the end of the waking period, and 'hates to get up in the morning' ...", who shows "a rising body temperature during the day," and whose performance (p 11) is better in the afternoon.

With respect to the establishment and maintenance of diurnal rhythms, he stated:

> "to take the human sleep-wakefulness cycle as an example of a fundamental metabolic variation of rest and activity, it is easy to follow the synchronization of this cycle with the 24-hour alternation of night and day in the life of a single individual. Practically from the day of birth, the baby is subject to 'acculturation' with the social environment, light, warmth, noise etc. ... impinging on it during the day. All of these stimulate activity, and thus metabolism, during a fixed fraction of the 24-hour period. Muscular activity raises body temperature, which increases the activity of the nervous system, the latter in turn augmenting muscular activity. In the older child and the adult there are established cortico-muscular circuits, or 'feed-back' mechanisms, to use the popular term, which operate like a vicious circle. Both muscular activity and nervous activity (metabolism, body temperature, efficiency of performance, etc.) keep rising. As the muscles get tired, not only from overt work, but from postural or tonic activity inherent in being awake, the trend is reversed. This reversal is aided by the onset of darkness, the lowering of air temperature, and the abatement of noises, characteristic of evening in the social routine of living. When the reversed trend of activity and metabolism has reached a certain low ('drowsiness level'), it becomes harder to remain awake. Sleep occasions a further drop in all the variables, until the diurnal minimum is reached ... Fundamentally, there is nothing about the sleep-wakefulness cycle that inherently demands a 24-hour spacing. Its synchronization with night and day is the easiest temporal adaptation for the organism to make, once the cortico-muscular circuits have been put into operation physiologically." (p 25-26) (Kleitman 1949b).

Finally in 1949, in a continuation of his study regarding the scheduling of working shifts in rotation (Kleitman, 1943), Kleitman (1949c) studied rest-activity cycles in submarine personnel. "One aspect of the problem of sleep aboard submarines is related to habitability and resolves around the space and comfort of sleeping accommodations. However, there is the much wider conception of sleep as one phase of the sleep-wakefulness cycle, which touches upon emotional stability and adjustment, as well as efficiency in performing the many different tasks assigned to the submarine personnel. The sleep-wakefulness cycle is more closely related to the problems of human engineering than those of habitability …" (p 329).

In the U.S.S. DOGFISH (SS350), there were three watch sections. Section I had the 4:00-8:00 and 16:00-20:00 watches. Section II had the 8:00-12:00 and 20:00-24:00 watches. Section III had the 0:00-4:00 and 12:00-16:00 watches.

On a 24-hour cycle, Kleitman suggested: For section I, watches 8-10, 12-16, 20-22. Sleep 22-6. For section II, watches 16-20, 22-24, 3-5. Sleep 6-14. For section III, watches 0-3, 5-8, 10-12 and sleep 14-22. The advantages of this suggestion for the concerns of the present article are that "hours of sleep may be optional, falling within the long stretches of free time available under all routines; the hours may also be fixed and … non–overlapping, permitting the exclusion of non-sleepers from sleeping quarters and the use of rotary bedding equipment" (p 337).

Kleitman also suggested "the possible advantages of a frank 12-hour cycle of wakefulness and sleep". With section I: watches 0-4, 12-16. Sleep: 6-10, 18-22. Section II: watches 4-8, 16-20. Sleep: 10-14, 22-2. Section III: watches 8-12, 20-24. Sleep 2-6, 14-18. "Hours of sleep may be optional, falling equally in each of the two 8-hour stretches of free time between watches or falling predominantly within one of the two 8-hour periods. Hours of sleep may also be fixed at 4 hours in the middle of each 8-hour period of wakefulness, permitting the exclusion of non-sleepers from sleeping quarters and the use of rotary bedding equipment … The criterion of superiority of the 12-hour cycle over the present skewed 24-hour one would have to be similar sleep-wakefulness and body temperature curves for all successive 12-hour periods" (p 339) (Kleitman 1949c). The author also suggested studies into cycles of longer than 24 hours for submarine personnel.

Following up on his previous research (Kleitman and Ramsaroop, 1948), Kleitman and Jackson (1950) studied mouth temperature and variations in performance speed and accuracy on a Link Trainer during the day and night in nine male subjects under different modifications of duty time. Sleep properties were not particularly taken into account, as the research mostly focused on the same topic as his earlier paper (Kleitman and Ramsaroop, 1948), addressing workers' schedules (Kleitman, 1943). The consequences of six different schedules were studied in the nine subjects as compared to in two controls, with performance being best when the body temperature was the highest. The smaller the deviation was from the usual routine (duty from 8:00 to 12:00 and from 13:00 to 17:00), the better was the adjustment. No changes in the usual diurnal body temperature curve occurred on a rotating activity routine ('involving daily changes in the hours of activity and sleep' (p 310)) … "The mean duration of sleep, under various activity schedules, did not deviate by more than half an hour from the control value of 8 hours, except that during one routine when the leisure hours were mainly in the forenoon, the mean duration of sleep was over 10 hours. During sleep the body temperature did not fall as low in the summer as it did in the spring, although the temperature and humidity of the air in the sleeping quarters were identical at all times." (p 328) (Kleitman and Jackson 1950).

Also in 1950, Kleitman participated in a symposium devoted to "Problems of consciousness" (Kleitman, 1950). Although the concept of consciousness is vast, it is necessary to expand on this topic to some extent here, because of the state of dreaming.

> "I don't like being obliged to set the tone for the term of 'consciousness' because I don't know exactly what it means. I feel it is a problem of semantics rather than physiology or psychology. However, I shall confine my remarks to what I call the garden variety of consciousness; that state in which we are supposed to be existing right now – in awareness of each other, of what we are saying, and of what is going on. This state is related to wakefulness and sleep in the sense that wakefulness, as we understand it in adult human individuals, implies a critical reactivity to one's environment … The definition of 'wakefulness' immediately breaks down when we consider the wakefulness of a newborn baby or decorticated mammal. You can tell when they are not asleep, but are they aware of what is going on? I doubt that. So, I shall speak of consciousness as related to wakefulness, and sleep, and it is one case where we can actually speak of level in the vertical sense. Some types of consciousness involved in dreaming, double personality, split personality, anesthesia, etc., may be really different types- different in kind rather than in degree" (p 15) …
>
> "I would call the lowest type of consciousness 'close to zero' the condition of a newborn baby when asleep. The next gradation, the condition of a newborn baby when awake, I like to call 'wakefulness of necessity' because it is really imposed upon the baby by conditions inside and outside its nervous system, its own body, a matter of getting fed, or being covered when it is cold, or uncovered when it is warm" (p 15).

The higher degree of "wakefulness of choice which in its rather primitive form is a low type of integration which does not involve a high degree of critical reactivity. This we find not only in the older baby who reaches for things, likes to play with things, smile at his mother, etc., but also in a sleeping individual who is dreaming" (p 16). Then, Kleitman spoke about performance and body temperature cycles, before a large discussion began on the floor regarding various topics related to wakefulness and sleep, and specifically addressing Bremer's, Magoun's and other researchers' neurophysiological results. As stated by Kleitman, "I want to say that I like being interrupted, so everyone should feel free to stop me or heckle me" (p 15), and indeed there were numerous interventions (paper of 45 pages). Indeed, concurrent to Kleitman's research between 1935 and 1950, other studies first showed the major importance of brainstem structures situated between the intercollicular level (Bremer 1935) and the medulla-medulla oblongata limit (Bremer 1936) for sleep and waking (Kerkhofs and Pevernagie 2012). Subsequently, the influence of this brainstem level was elucidated by stimulation (Moruzzi and Magoun 1949, Batini 2012) and lesion experiments (Magoun 1948, Lindsley et al. 1949, 1950) involving the midbrain reticular formation.

The diversity of Kleitman's fields of interest and his dynamism are surprising. In 1951, he and Engelmann published (Kleitman and Engelmann, 1951) a short communication reporting on a complete study of sleep in infants, which was an enrichment of his previous paper (Kleitman, 1949b). The later research (Kleitman and Engelmann, 1951) gave rise to the following results.

> "From continuous actograms and protocols kept by their mothers on specially designed forms, the incidence and duration of sleep was followed in 19 infants, from the 3rd to the 26th week of life, under family home conditions. Even the earliest records revealed a diurnal disparity, the mean group duration of night sleep being 8.4 hours, as against 6.4 hours for day (usually 8 a.m.-8 p.m.). Up to the 12th week, the total duration of sleep was unchanged, or slightly increased, but the night portion rose to 10.1 hours, at the expense of a corresponding fall in day sleep. For the succeeding 14 weeks, the duration of night sleep was unchanged, or slightly increased, but the day fraction continued to decrease, reaching 3.6 hours, for a total of 13.8 hours per 24 hours. Thus, not only were our objectively obtained figures much lower than those hitherto reported, but there was no marked diminution of sleep during the whole period of observation. The adjustment of the sleep-wakefulness pattern manifested itself mainly in a progressively more pronounced diurnal periodicity, culminating in one long unbroken period of night sleep and short morning and afternoon naps." (p 73-74) (Kleitman and Engelmann, 1951).

The next paper, also from 1951 (Kleitman and Schreider, 1951), was devoted to oculomotor performance (blinking rate, binocular fixation and lateral oscillation of the eyes) in 13 men and 5 women who were kept awake for about 30 hours. Sleep amount was not taken into account; only results that were altered due to drowsiness were reported.

> "Poorest performance occurred in the early hours of the morning, coinciding with the development of drowsiness … Without intervening sleep, there was a spontaneous recovery of oculomotor performance, along with an increase in alertness, later in the morning or afternoon … Amphetamine had no effect on oculomotor performance of subjects when the subjects were wide-awake, but led to improvement of impaired performance observed during drowsiness. Small amount of alcohol often imitated the impairment of oculomotor performance that occurred in drowsiness." (p 214).

In a short communication, Kleitman (1952) reported a study in which "during the continuous daylight of the arctic summer, at Tromso, in Norway, a family of 3 women and 1 man followed artificial sleep-wakefulness schedules, with appropriate adjustments of activity and meal hours. First, an 18-hour routine was adhered to for 3 weeks, then there were 2 weeks of 'normal' living, followed by 3 weeks on a 28-hour routine. Each artificial schedule necessitated sleeping around the clock, but the depressing effect of having, at times, to carry on 'daytime' activities in the dark was absent. The new routine curve disrupted the regular diurnal temperature curve of the women, but … definite 18- and 28-hour curves were not developed. The man … showed … a complete fixity of the 24-hour body temperature curve on both the 18- and 28-hour schedules. By contrast, the heart rate … promptly conformed to the 18- and 28-hour routines, acquiring distinct new curves. It thus appears that the diurnal body temperature curve is a rhythm not easily modified by a change in routine, whereas the quite parallel heart rate curve would seem to be a simple periodicity, immediately determined by the particular schedules of hours of sleep, activity, and meals." (p 83).

The next paper (Kleitman and Esther Kleitman, 1953) was the full report of the previous short communication (Kleitman, 1952). It revealed that the subjects described in the earlier communication were Kleitman, his wife, and their two daughters (Esther and Hortense), who migrated to Norway from May 21 to July 23, 1951 to perform this experiment; the paper was published together with Esther.

> "Two 3-week periods of artificial living routines, one of 18 and the other of 28 hours, were separated by 2 weeks on the usual 24-hour schedule … The 18-hour routine called for 6 hours of sleep and 12 of

wakefulness with two meals during the latter … The 28-hour schedule allowed 8-9 hours of sleep and 20-19 of wakefulness, with three meals, spaced somewhat wider than usual … Subjectively, the 18-hour routine was more acceptable than the 28-hour one, probably because the 'turn-over' interval in the former was only 3 calendar days (4 x 18 hours), whereas in the latter it was a whole week (6 x 28 hours)." (p 284).

In addition to the temperature and heart rate described in the previous paper, motility was also studied during sleep by actograms, during quiescent periods of quarter-hour duration and multiples thereof and "the counter readings of summated displacement of the recording lever varied of summated displacement varied directly with motility" (p 285).

"Adherence to 18-hour and 28-hour sleep-meal-activity schedules … under continuous daylight … led to a disruption of the usual diurnal oral temperature rhythm in Esther and Hortense, but not in Kleitman . By contrast, the heart rate observed in two subjects (including the temperature-fast one) promptly conformed to the two non 24-hours routines by acquiring distinct 18-hour and 28-hour periodicities» (p 291) (Kleitman and Kleitman, 1953).

Also in 1953, Kleitman and his daughter Hortense (Kleitman and Kleitman, 1953) studied sleep-wakefulness patterns in arctic inhabitants who "are apt to sleep only three or four hours a day during the summertime". The study was performed in Tromso, situated about 200 miles north of the Arctic Circle. "The sun describes a daily circle in the sky, remains above the horizon from May 21 to July 23" (p 350). The authors described, in detail, the local life led by the inhabitants during the summertime. The research involved interviews (49 males, 51 females), addressing the times at which they go to bed and get up, and the duration of their sleep during the winter, in the absence of any daylight, and during the summer. (Figure 20).

"The data on the sample of the inhabitants of Tromso, Norway, where the sun does not set during the summer and where continuous darkness prevails during the winter, show only a slight deviation from the sleep-wakefulness pattern that characterizes the diurnal routine in living in civilized communities in middle latitudes, and incidentally reveal that an average of 7 hours of sleep per night is probably compatible with the maintenance of well-being in human adults" (p 356).

In this paper there is a photo of Kleitman and Hortense at the sea side near a whale (Figure 21) (Kleitman and Kleitman, 1953).

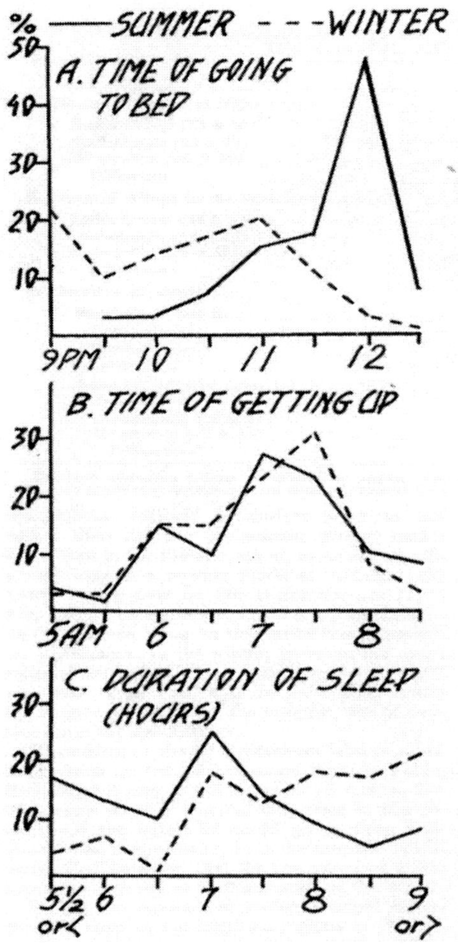

Figure 20. Sleep in the Arctic Circle. "The data on the sample of the inhabitants of Tromso, where the sun does not set during the summer and where continuous darkness prevails during the winter, show only a slight deviation from the sleep-wakefulness pattern that characterizes the diurnal routine in those living in civilized communities in middle latitudes, and incidentally reveal that an average of seven hours of sleep per night is probably compatible with the maintenance of well-being in human adults" (p 356). Reprinted from *Scientific Monthly.*

Again in 1953, Kleitman and Engelmann (1953) published a full paper which followed up on their short report from two years earlier (Kleitman and Engelmann 1951). It concerned sleep characteristics in infants. A beautiful figure best summarizes their results on the appearance of a sleep-waking cycle in a young girl (Figure 22).

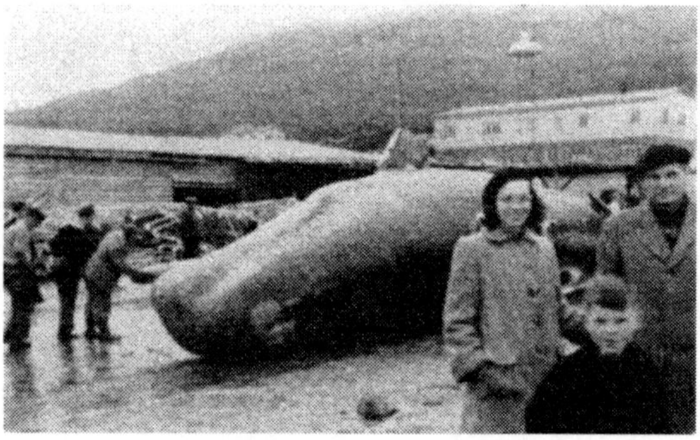

Figure 21. The authors with a young friend at a Tromso (Norway) whale-processing yard. Reprinted from *Scientific Monthly*.

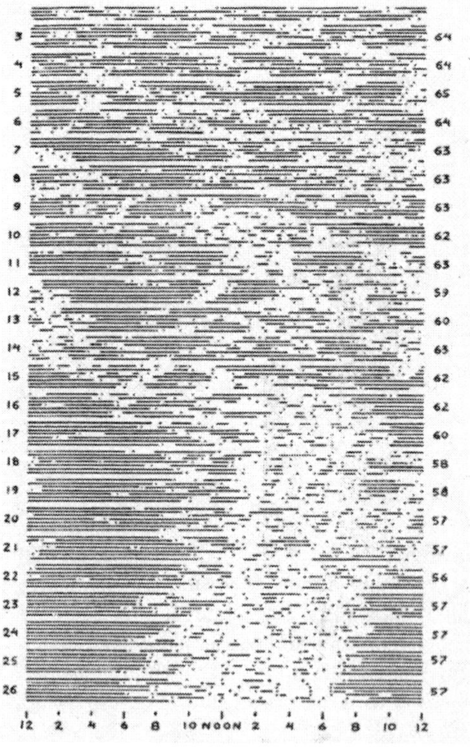

Figure 22. Ontogenetic progressive appearance of a structured sleep-waking cycle. The infant was studied from the 11th to the 182th day. Dark bands are sleep periods, the breaks between the black lines represent waking and the dots, feeding. The successive weeks are shown on the left, the percentage of sleep during the successive weeks appears on the right column, and the time, in 2-hourly intervals, is shown at the bottom. Reprinted from *Journal of applied Physiology.*

"It was a first baby and its parents were sufficiently indulging to permit it to set its own sleep-wakefulness and feeding schedule. The top and the bottom of Figure 22 in which the progress of this infant is shown, do not differ from any other infant's chart. They show an initial haphazard distribution of sleep and feedings and a terminal adjustment to an uninterrupted 10-hour during sleep during the night (8 p.m. to 6 a.m.), short naps and feedings during the intervening hours." (p 276).

"For the several infants observed, the rate of activity at the onset of sleep decreased gradually, though not always steadily, to zero … Eye movements gradually subsided during the change from wakefulness to sleep. The complete cessation of ocular movement (as seen directly) lasted for a less variable period, which was approximately 23 minutes for the several infants observed. On the basis of eye movements alone, awakening appeared to be more abrupt than the onset of sleep …

… The afternoon naps or long night sleep stretched of these infants were not homogenous, but appeared as rest-activity cycles which had a duration of considerable range, with a mean value of about 1 hour … At night, the infants generally proceeded from one cycle to the next without any great outburst of activity." (p 281).

It is of interest to mention that, first, Kleitman had thus already probably observed eye movements during sleep (directly under the eyelids) in 1951, although this analysis had not been mentioned in the preliminary paper. Second, in a footnote he thanked 'Mr Eugene Aserinsky' for the detection of eye motility and "for the analysis of actograms that led to the detection of the fundamental hourly periodicity" (p 281) Kleitman and Engelmann (1953).

The famous discovery of REM sleep also occurred in 1953. Although several premonitory results had been published earlier (for ref. see (Gottesmann, 2001, Schulz and Salzarulo 2012), this year is retained for its definitive identification. To follow the historical steps, we must start with a short commentary on eye movements occurring during sleep that was published by Aserinsky and Kleitman (1953a) in March of that year.

"Electro-oculograms and electroencephalograms were recorded by means of a Grass Electroencephalograph on 12 normal male adult subjects during sleep. Eye movements were distinguished from brain wave artifacts by the greater amplitude of the corneo-retinal potential in the electro-oculogram in contrast to the height of the potential on a unipolar lead near the eye. Rapid eye movements, indicated by potentials of up to 300 microvolts, were observed to appear from 2 to 5 h (3.8 h mean) after the onset of sleep in 10 subjects. The concurrent occipital brain wave pattern was, in all cases, indicative of drowsiness or very light sleep. This was confirmed by the subject's failure to respond to an auditory stimulus of above waking threshold intensity. There is a very strong suggestion that these eye movements occurring during sleep are associated with dreaming. The duration of this eye movement pattern may be a half minute or less. More frequently, the pattern persisted until the artificial interruption of sleep at the end of the 2 minute period. Upon resumption of sleep, the eye movements frequently reappeared as often as four times within a half hour." (p 6-7).

The full paper appeared in Science on September 4th. (Aserinsky and Kleitman 1953b).

"Slow, rolling or pendular eye movements such as have been observed in sleeping children or adults (by four mentioned authors) have also been noted by us. However, this report deals with a different type of eye movement –rapid, jerky and binocularly symmetrical- which was briefly described elsewhere (p 273) ... (see above Aserinsky and Kleitman 1953a).

... The eye movements were recorded quantitatively as electro-oculograms by employing one pair of leads on the superior and inferior orbital ridges of one eye to detect changes of the corneo-retinal potential in a vertical plane, and another pair of leads on the internal and external canthi of the same eye to pick up mainly the horizontal component of eye movement." (p 273).

"... To confirm the conjecture that this particular eye activity was associated with dreaming, 10 sleeping individuals in 14 experiments were awakened and interrogated during the occurrence of this eye motility and also after a period of at least 30 min to 3 hr of ocular quiescence... Of 27 interrogations during ocular motility, 20 revealed detailed dreams usually involving visual imagery; the replies to the remaining 7 queries included complete failure, or else, 'the feeling of having dreamed' but with inability to recollect any detail of the dream. Of 23 interrogations during ocular inactivity, 19 disclosed complete failure of recall ... The ability to recall dreams is significantly associated with the presence of the eye movements noted, with a X^2 p value of less than 0.01." ... (p 273-274).

"... The first appearance of a pattern of rapid, jerky eye movements was from 1 hr 40 min to 4 h 50 min (3 h 14 min mean) after going to bed ... The period from the onset of the first recognizable pattern to the disappearance of the last pattern was from 6 to 53 min with a min of 20 min. A second period of eye patterns appeared from 1 h 10 min to 3 h 50 min (2 hr 16 min mean) after the onset of the first eye motility period. With lengthier sleep there occurred a third and, rarely, a fourth such period ... (Simultaneous) recorded monopolar EEG's from the frontal and occipital areas ... were invariably of low amplitude (5-30 μV) and irregular frequency (15-20/sec and 5-8/sec predominating)."... (p 274).

"... In another series of experiments involving 14 subjects, the respiratory rate was calculated for a minimum of ½ min during eye motility and compared with the rate for a similar duration 15 min before and after an eye motility period. The respiratory rate had a mean of 16.9/min during eye motility in contrast with 13.4/min during eye quiescence ... Fisher's t method: p less than 0.001. Experiments now in progress suggest that heart rate also is probably higher in the presence of these eye movements ... In every case the eye motility periods were associated with peaks of overt bodily activity although the latter were frequently present in the absence of eye movements." (p 274) (Figure 23).

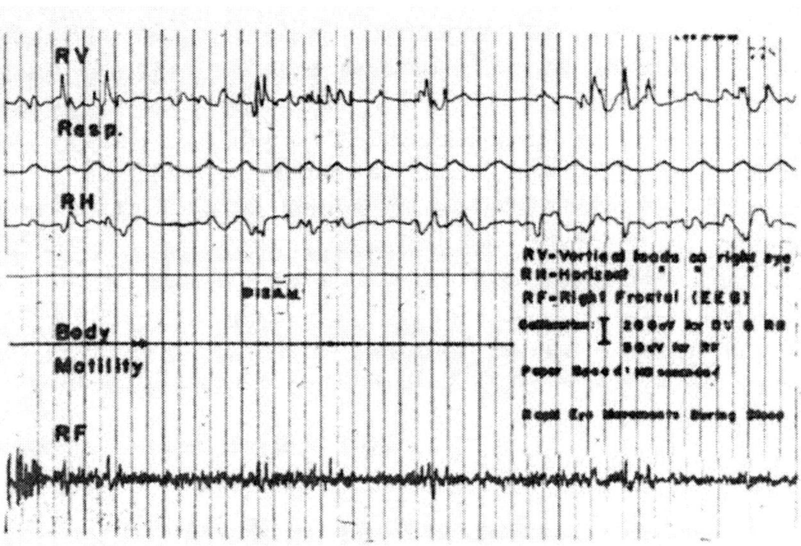

Figure 23. REM sleep recording. RV and RH, vertical and horizontal recording of eye movements. Res, respiration. RF, right frontal EEG recording. Reprinted from *Science*.

... The fact that these eye movements, EEG pattern, and autonomic nervous system activity are significantly related and do not occur randomly suggests that these physiological phenomena, and probably dreaming, are very likely all manifestations of a particular level of cortical activity which is encountered normally during sleep. An eye movement period first appears about 3 h after going to sleep, recurs 2 h later, and then emerges at somewhat closer intervals a third or fourth time shortly prior to awakening. This method furnishes the means of determining the incidence and duration of periods of dreaming." (p 274) (Aserinsky and Kleitman 1953b).

This fundamental and very precise description of REM sleep calls for a short commentary, in view of a paper published in 1996 (Aserinsky, 1996). Surprisingly, Aserinsky's paper was written 43 years after the discovery of REM sleep. Why so late, when Kleitman, at the age of 101 years, was probably no longer able to confirm or criticize its content? Moreover, it is known that memories are often subject to modification with time. Forty-three years was also the latency of Maury's report of his famous, and questionable, instantaneous dream during which he was ill, with his mother sitting at his bed side (Maury, 1861) (translation Gottesmann, 1999). It is difficult to believe that Kleitman, as related by Aserinsky, only "had a tangential role in my REM project" (p 222); indeed, in 1968, prior to any controversy, Bernadine Lufkin (1968) had written "I was not present when Dr. Aserinsky came to Dr. Jacobson, at the request of Professor Kleitman, to learn how to record eye movements during sleep. I understand that he was told that Dr. Jacobson had developed these methods and described them in his book on sleep" (p 449). The description and quotation of Jacobson's findings about eye movements and dreaming can be found in Kleitman's book (Kleitman, 1963) (p 94) and in (Gottesmann, 2001). Lufkin further stated "I have a photostat of a letter dated June 15, 1961, written to Dr. Jacobson by Dr. Aserinsky ..." Years had to pass before your conversation made the deepest impact ... I would like you to know that you have my deepest respect for your pioneer contributions in physiology and psychology." (p 449). This first sentence suggests that, in those days, Aserinsky was a following fellow, rather than the initiator of the idea to go to learn Jacobson's method. The assertion of the 'tangential' role of Kleitman is the most open to question, since Kleitman (see above in 1939) had already clearly observed rapid EEG periods during which dreaming occurred (Blake et al., 1939); this had already been shown in 1937 (Loomis et al., 1937). Finally, Aserinsky said that Kleitman, unaware and doubtful of the result of this experiment, required that one of his daughters be a control subject. As noted above, Esther Kleitman, who, like her sister Hortense, was a co-author of certain of her father's papers, did not confirm this assertion (personal communication, February 2012). As written previously (Gottesmann, 2001), Aserinsky told me once in the seventies that when he defended his thesis at Chicago University in 1953, the examiners told him that doctorates are rewarded not for obtained findings but in the hope of future results. He was a fellow of the National Institute of Mental Health when he undertook this research, which gave rise to his first published result. Personally, perhaps based on a misunderstanding, I think that in his 1996 paper Aserinsky somewhat underestimated Kleitman's contribution.

The next paper (Aserinsky and Kleitman, 1955a) was devoted to a more precise analysis of the appearance of the slow and rapid eye movements that occur during sleep.

> "The ocular motility curve was based on the continuous EOG (electrooculogram) as well as from direct observations of the lids for one or more minutes during approximately each successive 5 minutes" (p 4) …
>
> "Slow eye movements were seen at the onset of sleep and together with and after every body movement throughout sleep" (p 3) …
>
> "The EEG during the long periods of ocular quiescence revealed delta waves or definite 12-14/sec. spindles or a combination of both. Although eye movements were never observed in the presence of a predominant delta pattern, some slow eye movements were occasionally seen concurrent with 14/sec. spindles which appeared outside of these long periods of ocular inactivity." (p 4) …
>
> "… From 1 to 5 hours (average 3 h) after the onset of sleep, the first group of rapid eye movements appeared simultaneously in both eyes. They persisted for a variable duration, disappearing and then reappearing, until about 20 minutes later the last cluster of movements could be discerned. After 2 hours of ocular quiescence (including slow eye movement) there usually occurred another period of rapid eye movement which did not differ significantly in duration from the first period. Again, about $1_{1/2}$ hours later, a third period of such movement sometimes appeared. With longer sleep, a fourth period of eye movement appeared." (p 4).

This was the first identification of the 90-minute cycle of REM sleep appearance. "The rapid eye movement periods appeared concurrently with a low voltage brain wave pattern, but the latter was not always accompanied by the eye movements" (p 4), which never occurred during delta activity.

> "… The mean respiratory rate increased approximately 20% (during the eye movement periods), and this was significant at the 0.001 level of probability … The mean heart rate during the presence of the eye movements … was approximately 10% higher than in the control periods." (significant 0.001 level) (p 5).

Finally, Figure 24 clearly shows that there were more body movements (now most often called jerks) during the rapid eye movement periods.

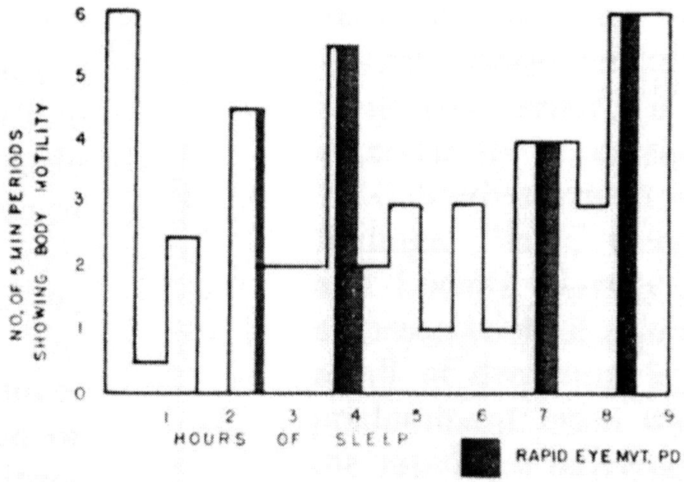

Figure 24. Relationship of body motility and rapid eye movements during sleep. The vertical bars represent the degree of body movements. Black areas indicate the occurrence of rapid eye movements. Reprinted from *Journal of applied Physiology*.

With respect to dreaming, to confirm that the subjects were indeed asleep during the low voltage cortical activity that was associated with the rapid eye movements, Aserinsky and Kleitman exposed them to an auditory stimulus above the waking threshold.

> "The recall of dreaming was associated with the prior occurrence of rapid eye movements at a probability level of less than 0.01." (p 6) …
>
> "… No sex differences with respect to the ocular activity and concomitant phenomena were noted in this study. Rapid eye movements appeared in the child and were apparently no different from that seen in adults. ... However, there was the suggestion that the child's slow eye movement and body motility behavior bore a closer resemblance to the regularity of the rest-activity cycles than did the adult pattern." (p 7) (Aserinsky and Kleitman, 1955a).

The notion of "rest-activity cycle" thus entered into Kleitman's body of work.

The same year, the next paper (Aserinsky and Kleitman, 1955b) concerned infant sleep "to determine what relationship the motor activity of the extraocular and palpebral musculature has to the occurrence of overt body movements, and consequently to the depth of sleep" (p 11). The observations, made at home, were performed on 14 infants of from 1 to 7 months of age.

"Except for three observations conducted during the night, the studies were performed in the morning or afternoon" (p 11). Eye and eyelid movements were visually determined and inscribed by a mark upon a slowly moving tape, like the body movements detected by a mechanical leverage device. Figure 25 shows that during the eyeball or lid movement periods there were also body movements, although "no so evident from the graph is the observation that ocular motility away persisted for a short while after the cessation of all discernible movement." (p 12).

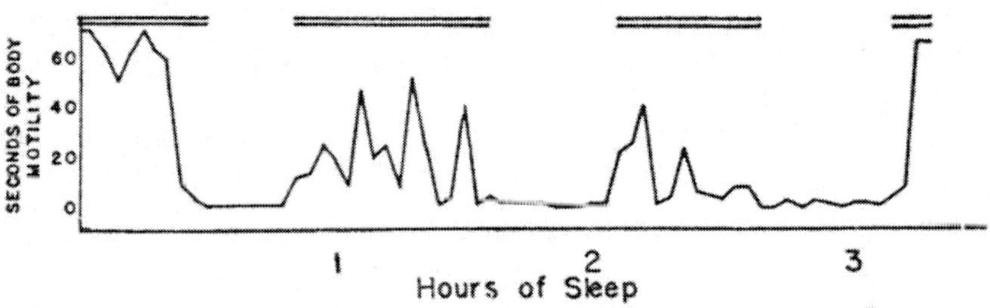

Figure 25. "Relationship of ocular activity to body movement during the sleep of an infant. The *Solid line* represents a quantitative measure of body movement. The d*ouble bar* indicates lid or eyeball movement and breaks in the double bar represent intervals of complete absence of observable ocular motility" (p 12). Reprinted from *Journal of applied Physiology.*

> … "Whereas the No Eye Movement period was characterized by its relative constancy, the active period of the motility cycle tended to be altered by age, time of day and, of course, tremendous individual differences. For seven infants (of our own observation) the means of the entire motility cycle ranged from 37 to 96 minutes in contrast with 19 to 26 minutes means for the No Eye Movement periods … The infant sleeps for one motility cycle (approximately 1 hour) and then stirs abruptly either to return to sleep for the duration of another motility cycle or else to remain awake until its demands (for example feeding are satisfied) (p 18) … The etiology of the motility cycle remains unresolved in the absence of additional experimental findings (p 17) … As possible sources of stimulation affecting the observed rest-activity cycle in infants, one cannot overlook the stimulation from the periphery due to lying in one position as well as the possibility of an inherent rhythm within the CNS." (p 18) (Aserinsky and Kleitman, 1955b).

Still in the same year, in March, Kleitman's first paper in collaboration with William C. Dement appeared (Dement and Kleitman, 1955). This short communication was devoted to the relationship of sleep-related eye movements and EEG.

> "Extending earlier observations on rapid eye movements, probably connected with dreaming (Aserinsky and Kleitman. Science 118 ; 273, 1953), in 16 male subjects (43 subject-nights) such movements were found to be associated with an individually characteristic low-voltage EEG, randomly irregular, without spindling. Calling this least constant sleep pattern Stage 1, a flatter low-voltage EEG, with spindling, stage 2, delta waves exceeding 100 microvolts, with spindling, stage 3, and half-or-more high voltage activity, stage 4, one could discern a succession of 60-80-min. swings in EEG pattern, with a progressive decrease in maximum, as well as in amplitude, during a single night's sleep. Composite histograms of the frequency distribution of rapid eye movements and of the swings in the continually recorded sleep EEG stages showed that in the first 6 hr. of sleep the peaks of eye movement episodes coincided with the minima of these swings, and that the duration of eye motility increased with the progressive lowering of the maxima of the swings. The mean lengths of successive episodes were 8, 16, 22 and 24 min. In spite of individual and group variation in the phenomena studied, there was an overall regularity in the repetitive swings in the EEG pattern and the interspersed periods of eye motility during a night's sleep." (p 37).

One comment can be made here: It is rather unexpected that the authors said that the rapid eye movements were 'probably' related to dreaming, coming after the four previous papers clearly demonstrating this relationship (Aserinsky and Kleitman, 1953a,b; Aserinsky and Kleitman, 1955b).

Finally, following his previous contribution (Kleitman (1950) at the first symposium devoted to Problems of Consciousness, Kleitman (1955) gave a new communication at the fifth Conference, concerning the function of the cerebral cortex in consciousness.

> "I am now convinced … that we shall deal with consciousness as something that may occur in wakefulness and in sleep, and that one can be awake and be non-conscious, and asleep and conscious … That is, a newborn baby, with due apology to anthropologists, in my view, is a decorticated animal. A decorticated dog or cat can wake up or sleep without any distinct evidence of consciousness, which, of course, brings us up against the definition of consciousness, which we have already found a very hard thing to formulate." (p 111) (see above Kleitman 1950).

The author then presented the different steps involved in the appearance of consciousness in babies, such as the recognition of their mothers' faces, i.e. discrimination among other faces. "Even in recognition there are different stages and different degrees of complexity" (p 112). Another characteristic that was underlined: the ability to recall, which necessarily involves both memory and the fact of having been conscious at the time when the recalled event occurred. For Kleitman, the first form of memory to develop "is sensory or analytical or differential ... Analysis comes first; integration afterwards" (p 112). Time is another important element: "you do something to meet a situation in the light of your experience, that is, for the present or for the future that is quite imminent." Then, he reported his recent findings related to consciousness during sleep in view of the discovery of REM sleep, related to the concept of the remembering of dreams. A very rich discussion followed, involving numerous contributors from the floor, regarding different topics such as wakefulness, degrees of consciousness ... The paper was 21 pages long; in the references, there was no mention of his own research.

In 1956, another short commentary by Dement and Kleitman (1956) was published concerning the relationship between rapid eye movement and dreaming.

As previously reported (Dement and Kleitman, 1955), EEGs obtained during sleep exhibit a series of successive variations, with discrete periods of rapid eye movements occurring during the 'lightest' phase of each cycle. In this later paper, Dement and Kleitman (1956) studied body motility in 20 subjects and dream recall in 2 subjects in relation to these variations.

> "Histograms revealed that body motility: 1) gradually decreased as sleep 'deepened' and then rose to a peak with the lightening of the EEG, decreasing again as the next cycle started; and 2) dropped sharply at the onset of the rapid eye movements, rebounding abruptly as the eye movements ceased. One subject gave a detailed description of dream content in 36 of 40 awakenings while the eyes were moving, and there was a general correspondence between the length of the reports and the duration of the eye movement periods. No dream recall was elicited after 26 awakenings at other times. The subject was awakened 21 times either 5 or 15 minutes after the eye movements had begun and judged the dream duration correctly each time. Findings in the second subject confirmed those of the first." (p 46).

This short abstract only confirmed and slightly enriched the previous results of Aserinsky and Kleitman. Either Dement was for the first time convinced by the previous results showing an association between rapid eye movements and dreaming, or was it, unexpectedly, Kleitman? It is worth pointing out that, the previous year, Dement studied eye movement periods and related dreaming activity in normal and schizophrenic patients ('treated' by prefrontal lobotomy!) (Dement, 1955). This abstract curiously was not mentioned in their later complete papers, in contrast to the 1955 short commentary (Dement and Kleitman, 1955).

Three papers were published in 1957. The relative order of the first two is difficult to establish, unlike the third which can be placed by its references. The first (Kleitman, 1957) was a major commentary on other authors' publications and was devoted to the distinction between sleep, waking, wakefulness and consciousness [it is partly the continuation of an idea that had been addressed twice before (Kleitman, 1950, 1955)]. In the first part of this paper, Kleitman recalled that while the brainstem reticular formation is involved in the maintenance of waking and the mesodiencephalic system is responsible for wakefulness, "the subcortical system ... should be designated as the 'wakefulness center' and not the 'waking center' as it is responsible for the maintenance of wakefulness and not merely for the phenomenon of arousal from sleep." (p 355). For example, the EEG is not a good index of wakefulness, since, particularly under atropine, slow wave EEG sleep patterns can be observed in behaviorally awake dogs (Wikler, 1952). Moreover, "phylogenetic development and ontogenetic maturation account for the alternation of the innate sleep and wakefulness" (p 356). The wakefulness-sleep ratio is described as 1:2 with a periodicity cycle of 50 to 60 minutes in infants, and of 2:1 with a periodicity of 80 to 90 minutes in adults. As long as the mesodiencephalic wakefulness system is related to the cortex, it can induce a wakefulness-associated EEG. If this relationship is severed, however, either pharmacologically, electrically, or surgically, there can be a dissociation: wakefulness can occur with slow wave sleep EEG patterns (after atropine), or behavioral sleep can occur without EEG (after decortication). Finally, still in this first part of the paper, Kleitman recalled that an EEG-behavior dissociation is naturally observed during REM sleep, with wakefulness-associated EEGs occurring during behavioral sleep. In addition, it should be mentioned that Kleitman referred to his short abstract published together with Dement (Dement and Kleitman, 1955), but not to what is now considered the central paper concerning the discovery of REM sleep (Aserinsky and Kleitman, 1953b).

The second part of the paper concerned "the question of the place of consciousness in the sleep-wakefulness dichotomy" (p 357)

> … "Like ice and water they can be distinguished from each other by simple inspection. The melting point of ice or freezing point of water correspond to the drowsiness level or intermediate stage between wakefulness and sleep. Liquid water may be near the freezing point or close to the boiling point, and so may alertness vary from semi-wakefulness to manic hyperactivity ('boiling mad'). Conversely, the depth of sleep, like the coldness of ice, may be close to the transition state or way down near coma. In consciousness the sleep-wakefulness dichotomy is absent. There is only one state, whose criteria are partly objective, but mainly subjective, the observer making only inferences … The level of consciousness is variable and, at any moment, is determined by the degree of one's ability to utilize his past and contribute to his future. In the newborn infant, or older anencephalous child, as in the decorticated dog or cat, the level of consciousness is close to, if not at, zero. Their responses to stimuli do not meet the criteria for consciousness. Yet they show definite alternation of sleep and wakefulness, of the innate type, to be sure" (p 358) (Kleitman, 1957).

Today, a primitive level of consciousness, or at least of reactivity, is attributed to the advanced fetus.

The first complete paper by Dement and Kleitman (1957a) was devoted to the relationship between REM sleep and dreaming.

> "Discrete periods during which eyes exhibited rapid movements were observed in all nine subjects every night they slept. These periods were characterized by low-voltage relatively fast patterns in the EEG. The interspersed periods in which rapid eye movements were absent showed EEG patterns indicative of deeper sleep, either a predominance of high voltage, slow activity, or frequent, well-defined sleep spindles with a low-voltage background. No rapid eye movements were ever observed during the initial onset of sleep although the EEG always passed through a stage similar to that accompanying the rapid eye movement" (p 340).

This last sentence seems to concern stage 1 of sleep onset, which has later been shown to correspond to sleep onset REM sleep (SOREM) (Foulkes and Vogel 1965, Takeuchi et al., 1999, 2001, Nielsen, 2000,), during which dreaming occurs without rapid eye movement (only with slow oscillating of the eyeballs). During desynchronized EEG occurring during sleep, "the eyes were not constantly in motion during such periods; rather, the activity occurred in bursts of one or two, up to fifty or a hundred movements … The average for the whole group (of Ss) was one REM period every 92 minutes" (p 340).

Then, the authors verified that dream recall upon induced awakening was highest during the eye movement periods (Table 10).

Table 10. Dream recall during REM sleep periods with and without rapid eye movements

S	Rapid Eye Movements		No Rapid Eye Movements	
	Dream Recall	No Recall	Dream Recall	No Recall
DN	17	9	3	21
IR	26	8	2	29
KC	36	4	3	31
WD	37	5	1	34
PM	24	6	2	23
KK	4	1	0	5
SM	2	2	0	2
DM	2	1	0	1
MG	4	3	0	3
Totals	152	39	11	149

Instances of dream recall after awakenings during periods of rapid eye movement or periods of No rapid eye movements. Reprinted from *Journal of experimental Psychology.*

> "The incidence of dream recall dropped precipitously almost immediately upon cessation of REM's ... When aroused during a deep stage of sleep characterized by high voltage, slow waves in the EEG, Ss often awoke somewhat bewildered ... Most of the instances of inability to recall dreaming after awakenings during REM periods occurred in the early part of the night" (p 342).

Then, the Ss were awakened 5 or 15 minutes after REM sleep period onset. The estimated duration of dreaming was generally correct, although they were only able to recall the latter fraction of dreams.

Finally, the authors looked for the correspondence between eye movements and dream content. After vertical movements "the dream involved a predominance of action in the vertical plane ... After 1 min. of little or no eye movement ... the dreamer was watching something" (p 344) (Dement and Kleitman 1957a). This last result was confirmed and extended some years later, partly with Dement's participation (Roffward et al. 1962) and by Herman et al. (1964).

It is of interest that although the references included one paper with Aserinsky from 1955 (Aserinsky and Kleitman 1955a), as well as his abstract with Dement from the same year (Dement and Kleitman 1955), and one paper by Dement alone (Dement 1955), Kleitman's major paper from 1953 about the discovery of REM sleep (Aserinsky and Kleitman 1953b), which already included a description of the primary results related to the topic, was not mentioned.

The next major paper was published in 1957 (Dement and Kleitman, 1957b). In contrast to the previous paper, which studied interrupted sleep occurring during rapid eye movement periods, this later paper examined sleep occurring during undisturbed nights. The sample of Ss was large (26 men and 7 women). The EEG, eye movements, body motility, and dreaming were analyzed over one or several nights. After recalling the different EEG night stages, the authors confirmed that there were no rapid eye movements occurring during descending stage 1, when there is rapid low voltage EEG, and that the eye movement periods, four on average, were longer lasting in the second part of the night, with their mean total duration being about 64 minutes.

> "The only pattern seen while the eyes were moving was stage 1 … The rapid eye movement periods occurred at regular intervals … termed cycles. The definition of the first cycle was from the onset of sleep to the end of the first eye movement period. The second was from the end of the first eye movement period to the end of the second and so throughout the night" (p 678-679).

The authors then described the evolution of sleep during the night, with the rapidly occurring stage 4 taking place after sleep onset, followed by the ascending stage 2, and then by stage 1 with rapid eye movements. During the night, stage 2 became predominant between the REM sleep periods, whose mean duration gradually increased (Figure 26).

With respect to the body movements occurring during sleep, the authors distinguished between major movements (changes in position of the whole body) and minor ones (usually stirrings and limb movements).

> "During stages 3 and 4, major movements were invariably accompanied by an upward EEG change which persisted for atleast a minute or two and …; often represented the upward swing of a cycle.

Minor movements were frequently, but not always accompanied by upward EEG changes. During stage 2, major movements usually resulted in a fleeting appearance of stage 1 or waking EEG while minor movements caused little apparent change and were usually followed by an immediate reappearance of spindling" (p 681).

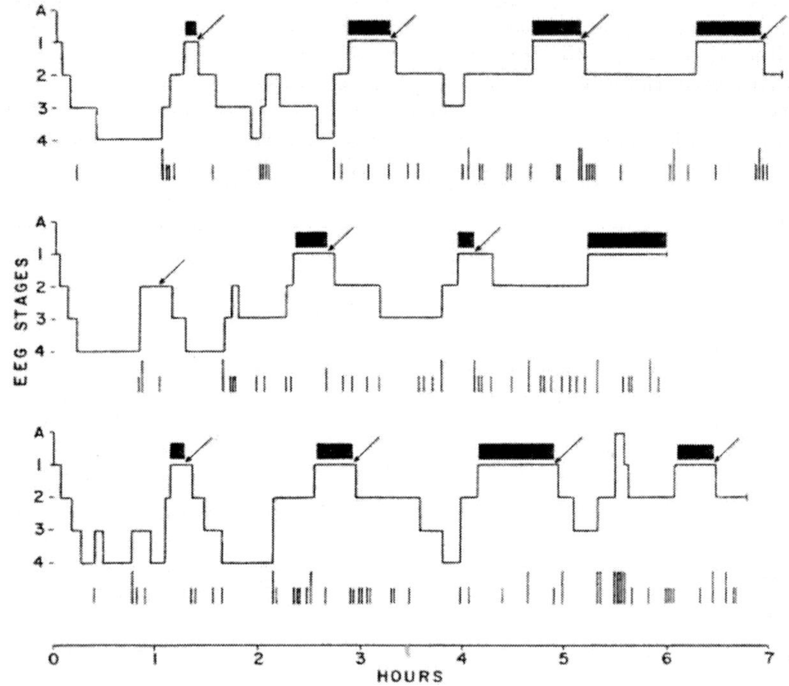

Figure 26. In three different subjects, the night begins with the rapid occurrence of stage 4. REM sleep (thick lines) is preceded by ascending stage 2. The duration of REM sleep periods increases during the night. Slow wave sleep becomes lighter as the night advances, as shown by the increased stage 2. The arrows show the end of each cycle and the beginning of the next one. Reprinted from *Electroencephalography and Clinical Neurophysiology*.

The authors then addressed the relationship between the body movements and the eye movements.

"During the actual experiment it was seen that rapid eye movement periods often started immediately after a series of body movements and that a body movement often coincided with their termination while the sleeper seemed relatively quiet during the eye movement period itself." (Figure 27)

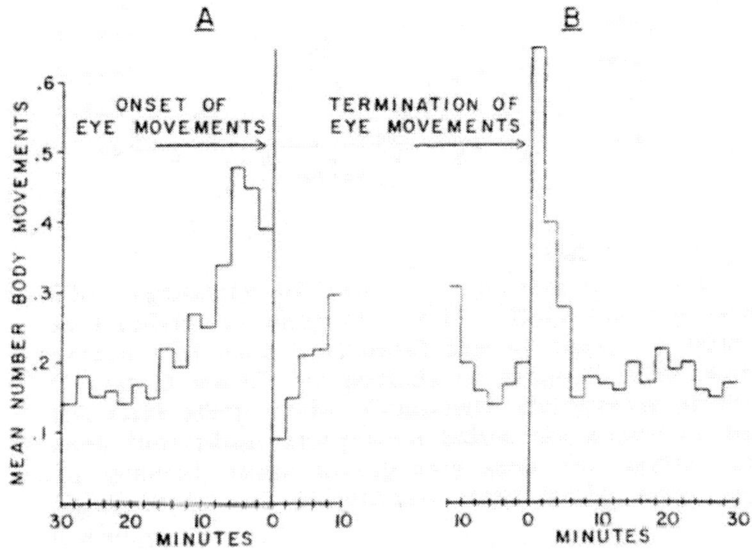

Figure 27. Relationship between gross body movements and rapid eye movements occurring at the onset (A) and termination (B) of REM sleep periods. The gross movements disappear during the REM sleep-associated rapid eye movements, and reappear at the end of REM sleep. Reprinted from *Electroencephalography and Clinical Neurophysiology*.

> "… Remembering that eye movements and stage 1 were concomitant … more body movements occurred while a stage 2 EEG was present than a stage 1 … During rapid eye movement periods numerous very small distal limb and digital movements occurred … which were almost entirely absent during the interspersed periods of ocular quiescence" (p 682). They had already been described in cats as "numerous jerks of single extremities" (p 514) (Klaue, 1937) (see Gottesmann 2001).

Then, stage 1 upon falling asleep was studied because of its absence of rapid eye movements. Their analysis showed that the mental content was "often 'dream-like' … distinctly different from actual dreams. (The subjects) invariably stated that they were not asleep and that the mental imagery was not as organized or 'real' as that occurring in dreams. A variety of images and sensations were described that might be called hypnagogic, such as 'floating', 'drifting', 'flashing lights' etc., … The later eye movement, stage 1, awakenings generally elicited dream recall and the impression of having been 'really asleep'" (p 683).

Finally, the auditory thresholds needed to elicit awakening from the subjects ranged from 0.1-0.4 at sleep onset and 1.0-1.8 during stage 1 ($P < .001$). The precise evaluation of the arousal threshold confirmed previous results (see above Mullin et al. 1937).

In the discussion, the authors recalled "with the exception of the initial onset of sleep, a persisting stage 1, non-spindling EEG seems to be invariably concomitant with dreaming while the amount of eye movement may be large or small depending on the actual imagery of the dream" (p 685).

The authors also discussed the previously-broached problem of consciousness during sleep (Kleitman, 1950, 1955, 1957). The discovery of REM sleep, enriched by the criteria of stage 1 EEG, modified the previous statements grounded in the activation of the brainstem reticular system, inducing waking and associated consciousness: "The ability to analyze, integrate, and subsequently recall experience … is not limited to wakefulness, nor does sleep always imply a very low or zero level of consciousness" (p 687). The mental activity taking place during sleep onset stage 1 ('hypnagogic reveries'), as well as during true REM sleep in established sleep, include the above characteristics of consciousness. "Behavioral criteria should take precedence in determining the presence of sleep or wakefulness, whereas the electroencephalogram may be more closely related to levels of consciousness" (p 689) (Dement and Kleitman, 1957b).

The next paper of Kleitman (1961), appearing soon before the major second edition of Sleep and Wakefulness (Kleitman, 1963) was devoted to the nature of dreaming. Presented at a symposium, it is a beautiful overview and synthesis of all of his own and his coworkers' results obtained since the discovery of REM sleep. Recalling the main properties of REM sleep (eye movements, EEG, heart pulses, respiration), he mentions the two 1955 papers written with Aserinsky, those co-authored with Dement, and other papers of Dement, but once again not the first, major 1953 paper. Concerning the eye movements, he recalls Ladd's observations (Ladd, 1892) (see Gottesmann, 2001) concerning their relationship to dreaming. The paper also addresses the increased responsiveness threshold that occurs during REM sleep, the issue of motility, the observation that the best recall of dreams takes place just after awakening and before evanescence, and the recall of dreams in schizophrenic patients, with 'isolated objects apparently hanging in space, with no movements' (Dement, 1955); in these patients Kleitman was thus "not in agreement with the idea that rapid eye movements are scanning movements" (p 358).

Kleitman postulated that the 80-90 minute interval between REM sleep episodes "is perhaps related to a primitive rest-activity cycle … This cycle is obscured during wakefulness by great surge of cortical activity, but suggestions of its presence may be discerned in daytime oscillations in alertness, the often irresistible drowsiness after a big meal, and the relief that some persons get from brief cat-naps" (p 361).

Ending with a discussion of the signification of dreaming, Kleitman stated that "A distinction should … be made between the phenomenon of dreaming and what one dreams about. Dreaming may be considered a rather uncritical cortical activity, with a short memory-span, associated with an emergent stage I EEG during sleep. Dream content is a secondary application of the primary dreaming process … Dream content, as a secondary application, may be of investigative or diagnostic interest to the psychologist or psychiatrist, may be a protection or disturbance of sleep, may or may not conform to Freud's views, but dreaming itself is probably a primary physiological process, associated with an emergent stage I EEG during sleep. The repetitive occurrence of dreaming in the course of a night's sleep, with its regularity of both incidence and duration, suggests that it is not initiated by sensory impulses, or by emotional tensions, but, like acquired sleep itself, of which it is a concomitant, depends on the development and functioning of a cerebral cortex for its manifestation" (p 363).

A discussion followed, involving Bremer, Eccles (the future Nobel Prize winner, in 1963), Jouvet, next leader in sleep research (Luppi 2012) as well as Dement, and others.

In 1967, Kleitman (1967a) studied the determinants of sleep-wakefulness cycles. He first centered his interest on the phylogenetic influences which specifically, in birds and mammals, affect the appearance of REM sleep (which occurs differently in different species), the duration of REM sleep episodes, and the latency between successive REM periods (which increases in conjunction with animal size). "A regular alternation of SWS and REM sleep characterizes the sleep EEG of all mammals investigated, and this physiological periodicity constitutes a basic rest-activity cycle (BRAC) – perhaps a fundamental variation in the functioning of the central nervous system, under neurohumoral control" (p 30). "The duration of the BRAC appears to be fairly constant, even though in adult man the (REM sleep) phase may increase ten-fold from the beginning to the end of a normal night's sleep" (p 30).

The author then gave examples from his own work as well as from the literature, stating that "the BRAC is probably operative also in wakefulness ("coffee breaks, catnaps, postprandial drowsiness").

The ontogenetic variations in REM sleep made it evident that the BRAC increases with age.

> "Sleep cycling is of 50-60 minutes in infants, 60-70 minutes in preschool children and 85-95 minutes in adult man" (p 31). At the same time, there is a decrease in the percentage of REM sleep (17% in lambs, 7% in sheep, 55% and then decreasing to 15% in rats, 55% to 80% in human neonates, 40% in older infants, 30% in preschool children, 18.5% in adolescents, 22% in young adults, and 13% to 18% in older adults). In contrast, "the wakefulness capability manifests itself also in the lengthening of single wakefulness periods... Slow to rise at first, wakefulness capability in Man eventually increases four-fold, as the sleep to wakefulness changes from 2:1 at birth to 1:2 at maturity" (p 32).

Studying the influence of the environment, Kleitman noted that: "that the 24-hour cycle is not a physiological necessity was shown by the prompt acquisition of rhythms longer or shorter than 24 hours, when an artificial schedule of hours of meals, activities and sleep was maintained for some days" (p 32). In the absence of any time cues, a 24 1/2-hour sleep-wakefulness periodicity rapidly appears. "It appears that the individual circadian periodicities, of unknown endogenous origin, are obscured by the establishment and maintenance of the customary 24-Hour sleep-wakefulness rhythm" (p 33).

The last part of the report concerned the evolution of consciousness. The alpha rhythm could be a criterion of cortical maturation. There is a gradual increase in frequency with age, prior to a reversal in old age "particularly in senile depression ... The level of consciousness may be related to the frequency of the alpha EEG pattern. When a certain degree of anatomical maturation and physiological performance has been reached, (REM sleep cortical EEG) leads-through cortical activation – to a crude type of consciousness which characterizes dreaming. Dreaming during this phase of sleep is as natural a consequence of cortical evolution as thinking is in wakefulness" (p 34).

A discussion on the floor followed (with Jouvet, Snyder and others), in which he concluded:

> "I don't take any stock in this so-called third type of being: I think we're either asleep or awake. And when we're asleep and when we're awake, we show the basic rest-activity alternations of higher and lower activity, this higher activity calling for action, and lower activity allowing us to rest from the action …
>
> … Now, it's of course a matter of opinion as to whether dreaming serves a function and whether it brings out this or that in the individual from his past life for use of the psychoanalysis. But we need not have any other explanation for dreaming than the appearance of a high frequency or low voltage activity" (p 38) (Kleitman 1967a).

Another paper on the BRAC was published the same year (Kleitman, 1967b), after already having been presented in another symposium in 1966; both of these had similar content to the previously analyzed paper. This latter 1967 manuscript noted that "the basic rest-activity cycle (BRAC) is a short-term periodicity in the functioning of the central nervous system of higher vertebrates" (p 2). Kleitman also recalled that the length of the cycle increases phylogenetically and ontogenetically. The paper was mostly concerned with REM sleep characteristics as indices of the BRAC. While the length of the BRAC for REM sleep occurrence, separated by SWS episodes, is stable, the duration of REM sleep episodes increases during the night: "Evidently the mechanism responsible for the BRAC is independent of the mechanisms which regulate the two phases" (p 2). Then, discussing the level of consciousness, he argued that it is of lower quality during dreaming than during waking: "The level of consciousness during dreaming may be likened to that of the very young child, the senile person, or the normal adult under the influence of a large dose of alcohol" (p 3). He noticed that tachycardia during sleep is an index of REM sleep occurrence, and that the eye movements "no doubt represent the scanning of the scene of action during dreaming in older children and adults" (p 3). Finally, concerning the arousal threshold, an index of central reactivity, it is high if the sound is meaningless to the subject, and low if the sound is meaningful, "particularly if it conveys the threat of punishment" (p 3) (Kleitman, 1967b).

In 1972, Kleitman (1972) opened the First International Congress of the Psychophysiological Study of Sleep with some introductory remarks. Aside from mentioning the different topics of the ten organized symposia, he underlined the "chicken-and-egg" type of studies devoted to elucidating if sleep is a cessation of wakefulness "or does sleep enable the organism to built up humoral agents depleted during wakefulness". Kleitman also suggested studies to clear up why the ratio of sleep to wakefulness is 2:1 at birth and 1:2

at maturity. Also "why does it take the neonate only 4 to 5 weeks to achieve an unbroken night's sleep, whereas a child must be 4 to 5 years old before unbroken wakefulness is maintained during the day?" (p 15).

In 1982, Kleitman (1982) undertook a review of the data concerning the BRAC "22 years later", his first mention of this concept having indeed appeared in 1961 (Kleitman, 1961) (see above). Carefully reviewing all of the available results of the literaure showing an ultradian cycle for eating, drinking, smoking, hand waving, perception performance, heart rate, pupillary diameter, motility, etc., Kleitman emphasized that during sleep, the BRAC is not only evidenced by the activity of the EEG and eye movements, but also by "gastric hunger contractions and sexual excitement – processes concerned with self-preservation and preservation of species - which led to the designation of the cycle as basic" (p 314). Concerning mental activity during sleep,

> "because of the low level of cortical function … perhaps related to a paucity of proprioceptive and other sensory stimulation - both analysis and integration are inferior to the performance of the waking brain. They may be likened to the quickly forgotten waking experiences of very young children, senile persons, and normal adults under the influence of an appropriate dose of alcohol. The highest cortical functioning often relates to projection of events into the future, and leads to act inhibition (8 of the 10 commandments begin with 'thou shalt not'), and the low level of cortical activity in dreaming often results in antisocial 'acts'" (p 314-315) …
>
> … "Dreaming, as cortical activity during the REM periods, is as inevitable in sleep as thinking is in wakefulness, and no particular function needs to be ascribed to it … Of course, the absence of a distinct purpose in dreaming does not preclude its utilization for diagnostic or therapeutic ends" (p 315) (remember previously Vaschide and Piéron, 1901a,b, 1902a). In humans, crying at first and speech later are applications of the expiratory phase of breathing, but that does not make phonation a function of respiration …
>
> … "The majority of investigators cited in this (his) review explicitly or implicitly supported, or found their data to be in accord with, the postulated operation of the basic rest-activity cycle in both sleep and wakefulness … The establishment of the 90-min NREM (SWS)-REM periodicity in human sleep led to the suggestion of the operation of a basic rest-activity cycle during both sleep and wakefulness, and, conversely, dreaming appears to be a component of the activity phase of the same periodicity during sleep, thus requiring no teleological explanation" (p 315) (Kleitman 1982).

Finally, this paper contained an exhaustive bibliography.

Kleitman's final paper that we found was a short commentary on the BRAC (Kleitman, 1993). It is a recollection of all of its available characteristics, in particular that it has a periodicity of 90 minutes, and that during sleep it is characterized "by deep sleep and a lighter activity phase. (This sleep) activity phase is represented by a brain wave frequency resembling that of wakefulness, an acceleration of respiration and heart rate, and contraction of the stomach, accompanied by rapid eye movements. Dreaming occurs during the activity phase. The BRAC has also been shown to be operative during wakefulness, with its activity phase involved in self-preservation via feeding and, at maturity, continuation of the species via reproduction" (p 65). This summary recalled that the sleep-to-wakefulness ratio changes from 2:1 to 1:2 from birth to maturation, and that the length of BRAC increases from 50-60 minutes in infancy to 85-95 minutes in adulthood. In the same way,

> "From birth on, wakefulness of necessity expresses itself in the need for nourishment, manifested by the hunger contractions of the stomach during the activity phase of the BRAC" ... With growth and development, in addition to wakefulness of necessity, a wakefulness of choice depends on the interests of the individual and environmental happenings or on there being 'something to do'. For instance ... gorillas in their natural habitat in the presence of an abundance of food generally spend only about 7 hours in wakefulness, with the remaining time devoted to 13 or 14 hours of night sleep and to several naps during the waking period. Similarly, a person left alone in the evening with little to do or otherwise bored may find it hard to keep awake, whereas the same individual, interested in what's going on at a party with friends, remains wide awake" (p 66).

Kleitman also presented again his previous demonstration that dreaming, during the activity phase of the BRAC in sleep, involves a lower level of critical reactivity in the cerebral cortex than the level observed in alert wakefulness. Thus, during dreaming, the level of consciousness may be compared to that of a very young child, a senile individual or a normal adult under the influence of a large dose of alcohol. Dream reports may be of value for diagnostic and therapeutic purposes, but dreaming, as a process, is as inevitable in the activity phase of the BRAC during sleep as thinking is in wakefulness ...

"… after the 90-minute sleep-dream cycle was discovered, it was proposed that this might be a basic rest-activity cycle operating around the clock, in wakefulness as well as in sleep, and this proposal was confirmed in several observational and experimental studies" (p 66). (Kleitman, 1993).

This paper seems to have been his scientific testament.

Chapter 8

Conclusion

The analysis covers Kleitman's successive papers during his incredibly long scientific career--from 1923 to 1993, or 70 years!- highlighting his tremendous contributions to the history of sleep research in the 20th century. Moreover, his two editions of *Sleep and Wakefulness*, published in 1939 and 1963, remain, along with Piéron's *Le Problème physiologique du sommeil*, the two major monographs on sleep of the past century. While the two editions of the book have the same eight, identically entitled chapters, the second edition is highly enriched relative to the first, as shown by the incredible increase in the number of references (4,337 references vs 1,434 for the first edition); this testifies to the remarkable progress made in studies devoted to sleep in general. Only considering references specifically concerned with REM sleep, from its discovery in 1953 up until 1965 (the publication date of the second edition), there were 317 publications; many of these publications came around the time of the book's appearance, with 67 published in 1964, 135 appearing in 1965, and 190 references published in 1966! (Gottesmann, 2005).

The eight parts of *Sleep and wakefulness* were successively devoted to: 1/ Functional differences between sleep and wakefulness, 2/ Course of events during the sleep phase, 3/ Periodicity, 4/ Interference with sleep and wakefulness, 5/ Spontaneous changes in the sleep-wakefulness rhythm, 6/ Means of influencing sleep and wakefulness, 7/ States resembling sleep and 8/ Theories of sleep. It can be noted that these two last parts have the same titles as in Piéron's *Le Problème physiologique du sommeil.*

The other most significant sleep-related publications of the 20th century were probably, first, the special issue of Ergebnisse der Physiologie, entitled *Neurophysiology and Neurochemistry of sleep and wakefulness*, with papers by Moruzzi (1963, 1972) (see Batini 2012) and Jouvet (1962, 1972) (see Luppi 2012), a book by Hobson (1988) and another one by Steriade and McCarley (1990). However, these major publications were devoted to more limited topics, while Piéron's thesis and Kleitman's two editions of *Sleep and Wakefulness* covered all areas of sleep research. There is no significant difference in the number of references between Piéron's thesis (1229) and Kleitman's first edition (again 1434), even though Kleitman included relatively few of Piéron's references («I shall dwell more on the new than on the old», p 6) (Kleitman, 1939); this attests to the fact that sleep research was already undergoing great advances during the second and third decades of the century. However, the second edition (Kleitman, 1963) once again reflects the extraordinary explosion of research after WWII, particularly with the development of EEG and the discovery of REM sleep.

Kleitman 'officially' retired in 1960, but as shown continued to publish at a high level.

He died in 1999 at the age of 104.

Chapter 9

General Conclusion

In this review, our aim has not been to directly compare Piéron's and Kleitman's research methods and findings, since a decade marked by extensive technical progress separated the end of the former's sleep-related work from the beginning of the latter's research; Kleitman, once again, clearly stated that the point of departure for his research was the end of Piéron's work (as reflected in his references, with the exception of his citations of Piéron's work). Moreover, and most importantly, Kleitman never replicated Piéron's research, but at most partly followed up on the latter's research topics. Our goal here has been rather to present a detailed overview of the work of both of these important scientists, to make the key writings of Piéron directly accessible to the English-speaking scientific community, and to pay homage to these two hugely talented sleep researchers from the last century. Whereas Piéron's sleep research covered only about 13 years out of his rich scientific career and explored major but limited topics of sleep processes, Kleitman devoted nearly his entire scientific career to the exploration of extremely varied aspects of sleep.

It is of interest that Piéron stopped his sleep studies in 1913, going on to publish in the following year an extensive article on sensory processes (the primary research focus of his career) (Piéron, 1914), again exactly ten years before Kleitman's first publication on sleep (1923). The latter highly appreciated the former's work, which was also performed both on Man and on dogs, and in *Sleep and Wakefulness* he very often refers to Piéron's results and "very illuminating discussion" (p 6) (Kleitman, 1939).

While Piéron only worked in France, Kleitman, just for his sleep studies, migrated to Scandinavia and even to the Arctic. Moreover, with his bright mind, he had also previously worked in Utrecht (Holland) for 6 months in 1923 (Kleitman and Magnus, 1924a,b; Kleitman and Kleijn de, 1924) on a totally different topic. Because of his high esteem for Piéron, Kleitman went to Paris to work with him directly after his stint in Utrecht; this collaboration gave rise to several co-authored papers devoted to vision (Kleitman and Piéron, 1924a, b; 1925, 1928). A later paper on the same topic followed in the United States (Kleitman and Blier, 1928). Later, he migrated to Bermuda for a short period, independent of his research on sleep, and published a paper on the diurnal variation of visual pigments in an isopod (Kleitman, 1940).

It is obvious that in view of his extremely rich body of research, performed either alone and or with the help of several assistants, his discovery of REM sleep, and his magnificent two editions of Sleep and wakefulness, Kleitman can certainly be considered the “Father of sleep research” of last century (Editorial 1999; Dement, 2001; Siegel, 2001). However, Piéron, when not working alone, was helped by only one colleague, and developed several complex methods to carry out a large body of original researches, primarily concerning the study of sleep mechanisms through the search for chemical sleep inducing factors. This research was ahead of its time, and raised issues that remain without definitive answers even today. Finally, in addition to this large body of work, in view of his highly remarkable *Le Problème physiologique du sommeil* he must be viewed as the pioneer of 20th century sleep research (Gottesmann 2012), and he was a constant reference for Kleitman as evidenced by the numerous quotations from Piéron in his papers and in the two editions of *Sleep and Wakefulness.*

Acknowledgments

I thank Dr. P. Follette for the translation of Piéron's quotations and for improving the English.

References

Ascrinsky, E (1996). The discovery of REM sleep. *Journal of History of the Neurosciences* 5:213-227.

Aserinsky, E., Kleitman, N (1953a). Eye movements during sleep. *Federation Proceedings* 12:6-7.

Aserinsky, E, Kleitman, N (1953b). Regularly occurring periods of eye motility, and concomitant phenomena during sleep. *Science* 118:273-274.

Aserinsky, E, Kleitman, N (1955a). Two types of ocular motility occurring during sleep. *Journal of Applied Physiology* 8:1-10.

Aserinsky, E, Kleitman, N (1955b). A motility cycle in sleeping infants as manifested by ocular and gross bodily activity. *Journal of Applied Physiology* 8:11-18.

Batini, C (2012). Giuseppe Moruzzi: an european school of neurophysiology in the university of Pisa. *European Sleep Research Society 1972-2012*, 40th Anniversary of the ESRS. Bassetti, CL, Knobl B, Schulz H. (Eds). Wecom Gesellschaft Kommünikation mbh & Co. Hildesheim: 69-70.

Bechterew, WM. (1913). *La psychologie objective*. Paris, Alcan (quoted by Littman)l

Benoit, O, Bloch, V (1960). Seuil d'excitabilité réticulaire et sommeil profond chez le Chat. *Journal de Physiologie* 52:17-18.

Berger, E, Loewy, R (1898). L'état des yeux pendant le sommeil et la théorie du sommeil. *Journal de l'Anatomie et de la Physiologie* 34: 364-418.

Berger, H (1929). Ueber das electroenkephalogram des Menschen. *Archiv für Psychiatrie und Nervenkrankheiten* 87:527-570.

Blake, H, Gerard, RW (1937). Brain potentials during sleep. *American Journal of Physiology* 119:692-703.

Blake, H, Gerard, RW, Kleitman, N (1939). Factors influencing brain potentials during sleep. *Journal of Neurophysiology* 2:48-60.

Bohn, G, Piéron, H (1906). Le rythme des marées et le phénomène de l'anticipation réflexe. *Comptes Rendus des Séances de la Société de Biologie* 61:660-661.

Bremer, F (1935). Cerveau "isolé" et physiologie du sommeil. *Comptes rendus des Séances de la Société de Biologie* 118:1235-1241.

Bremer, F (1936). Nouvelles recherches sur le mécanisme du sommeil. *Comptes Rendus des Séances de la Société de Biologie* 122:460-464.

Chauchard, P (1964). Henri Piéron et l'essor de la psychologie française. *Concours Médical* 5:6923-6927.

Claparède, E (1905). Esquisse d'une théorie biologique du sommeil. *Archives de. Psychologie* 4:246-349.

Cooperman, NR, Mullin, FJ, Kleitman, N (1934). Studies on the physiologie of sleep.XI. Further observations on the effects of prolonged sleeplessness. *American Journal of Physiology* 107:589-593.

Cruchet, R, Moutier, J. Calmette, A (1917). Quarante cas d'encéphalomyélite subaiguë. *Bulletin de la Société de Médecine des Hôpitaux de Paris* 41: 614-616

Delczynski, (1875). *Virchow und Hirsch Jahresbericht* 1:248 (quoted by Piéron)

Dement, W (1955). Dream recall and eye movements during sleep in schizophrenic and normals. *Journal of Nervous and Mental Diseases* 122:263-269.

Dement, W (1958). The occurrence of low voltage fast electroencephalogram patterns during behavioral sleep in the cat. *Electroencephalography and Clinical Neurophysiology* 10:291-296.

Dement, W (2001). Remembering Nathaniel Kleitman. *Archives Italiennes de Biologie* 139:11-17.

Dement, W, Kleitman, N (1955). Incidence of eye motility during sleep in relation to varying pattern. *Federation Proceedings* 14:37.

Dement, W, Kleitman, N (1956). Body motility during sleep and dream duration recall. *Federation Proceedings* 8:46.

Dement, W, Kleitman, N (1957a). The relation of eye movements during sleep to dream activity: an objective method for the study of dreaming. *Journal of Experimental Psychology* 53:339-346.

Dement, W, Kleitman, N (1957b). Cyclic variations in EEG during sleep and their relation to eye movements, body motility, and dreaming. *Electroencephalography and Clinical Neurophysiology* 9:673-690.

Derbyshire, AJ, Rempel, B, Forbes, A, Lambert, EF (1936). The effects of anesthetics on action potentials in the cerebral cortex of the cat. *American Journal of Physiology* 116:577-596.

Durham, AE (1860). The physiology of sleep. *Guy's Hospital Reports* 6:149. (Quoted by Berger & loewy 1898).

Duval, M (1882). Sommeil. *Nouveau dictionnaire de médecine et de chirurgie pratique*. Paris, Baillière 33: 262-288.

Economo von, C (1917). Encephalitis lethargica. *Wiener Klinische Wochenschrift* 30:581-585.

Economo von, C (1928). Théorie du sommeil. *Journal de Neurologie et de Psychiatrie* 7: 437-464.

Editorial, (1999). Kleitman, father of sleep research. *The University of Chicago Chronicle* 19:1-2.

Fessard, A (1951). Henri Piéron. *L'Année Psychologique* 7-13.

Fontana, F (1765). *Dei moti dell'iride*. Lucca. Stamparia Jacopo Giusti.

Foulkes, WD, Vogel, G (1965). Mental activity at sleep onset. *Journal of Abnormal Psychology* 70:231- 243.

Fraisse, P (1965). Les dernières années d'Henri Piéron. *L'Année Psychologique* 65:1-4.

Fraisse, P (1970). French origins of the psychology of behavior; the contribution of Henri Piéron. *Journal of the History of the Behavioral Sciences* 16:111-119.

Freud, S (1900). *The Interpretation of Dreams*. London: The Hogart Press.

Garcia-Garcia, F, Acosta-Pefia, E, Venebra-Munoz, A, Murillo-Rodriguez, E (2009). Sleep-inducing factors. *CNS and Neurolological Disorders-Drugs Targets* 8:235-244.

Georgiade, C (1970). Eléments cybernétiques dans l'oeuvre d'Henri Piéron. *L'Année Psychologique* 70:161-177.

Golz, F (1892). Der Hund ohne Grosshirn. *Pfügers Archiv Gesellschaft für Physiologie* 51:570-614.

Gottesmann, C (2001). The golden age of rapid eye movement sleep discoveries. I. Lucretius-1964. *Progress in Neurobiology* 65:211-287.

Gottesmann, C (2005). *The golden age of rapid eye movement sleep discoveries. 1965-1966*. New York: Nova Science Publishers, Inc.

Gottesmann, C (2010). The development of the science of dreaming. *International review of Neurobiology* 92: 1-29

Gottesmann, C. (2012). Henri Piéron, the pioneer of 20th century sleep research. *European Sleep Research Society 1972-2012*, 40th Anniversary of the ESRS. Bassetti, CL Knobl B, Schulz, H. (Eds). Wecom Gesellschaft Kommünikation mbh & Co. Hildesheim: 63-64.

Guerrini, G (1900Delle minute modificazioni di struttura della cellula nervosa corticale nella fatica. *Rivista di patologia nervosa e mentale* 5:1-18. Quoted by Piéron (1912).

Hammond, WA (1880). On sleep. *Gaillard's Medical journal* 29, February, and (1870) *Journal of Psychological Medicine*, April. Similarly quoted by Manaceine (1894) and Piéron (1912).

Herman, JH, Erman, M, Boys, R, Peiser, L, Taylor, ME, Roffwarg, HP (1984). Evidence for a directional correspondence between eye movements and dreaming imagery in REM sleep. *Sleep* 7 52-63.

Hess, CW (2012). W.R. Hess and the Swiss school. *European Sleep Research Society 1972-2012*, 40th Anniversary of the ESRS. Bassetti CL et al. (Eds). Wecom Gesellschaft Kommünikation mbh & Co. Hildesheim: 67-68.

Hess Jr, R, Akert K, Koella W (1950). Les potentiels bioélectriques du cortex et du thalamus et leur altération par stimulation du centre hypnique chez le Chat. *Revue Neurologique* 83:537-544.

Hess, WR (1931). Le sommeil. *Comptes Rendus des Séances de la Société de Biologie* 107:1333-1364.

Hobson, JA (1988). *The dreaming brain*. New York, Basic books.

Ishimori, K (1909). The demonstration of intracerebral substances in sleep-deprived animals: sleep-inducing substances as the true cause of sleep. *Chuo Igakkai Zasshi* 84:1-47.

Ivy, AC, Schnedorf, JG (1937). On the hypnotoxin theory of sleep. *American Journal of Physiology* 119:342.

Jacobson, A (1930). Electrical measurements of neuromuscular states during mental activities. III. Visual imagination and recollection. *American Journal of Physiology* 95:694-702.

Jacobson, A (1938). *You Can Sleep Well. The ABC's of restful sleep for the average person*. New York, Whittley House.

Jouvet, M, Michel F, Mounier D (1960). Analyse électroencéphalographique comparée du sommeil physiologique chez le Chat et l'Homme. *Revue Neurologique* 103: 189-205.

Jouvet, M (1962). Recherches sur les structures nerveuses et les mécanismes responsables des différentes phases du sommeil physiologique. *Archives Italiennes de Biologie* 100:125-206.

Jouvet, M (1972). The role of monoamines and acetylcholine-containing neurons in the regulation of the sleep-waking cycle. *Ergibnisse der Physiologie* 64:166-307.

Khatami, R, Baumann, C, Bassetti, CL (2012). Von Economo and the hypothalamus. *European Sleep Research Society 1972-2012*, 40th Anniversary of the ESRS. Bassetti, CL, Knobl B, Schulz H. (Eds). Wecom Gesellschaft Kommünikation mbh & Co. Hildesheim: 61-62.

Kerkhofs, M, Pevernagie, D. (2012). Frédéric Bremer 1892-1982: his "cerveau isolé" and "encéphale isolé" preparations. *European Sleep Research Society 1972-2012*, 40th Anniversary of the ESRS. Bassetti CL, Knobl B, Schulz H (Eds). Wecom Gesellschaft Kommünikation mbh & Co. Hildesheim: 69-70.

Klaue, R (1937). Die bioelektrische Tätigkeit der Grosshirnrinde im normalen Schlaf und in der Narkose durch Schlafmittel. *Journal für Psychologie und Neurologie* 47:510-531.

Kleitman, N (1923). Studies on the physiology of sleep. I. The effects of prolonged sleeplessness on man. *American Journal of Physiology* 66:67-92.

Kleitman, N (1924). Beitrage zur pharmakologie der Koerperstellung. XII Mitteilung. Ueber der Wirkung von Atropin und Pilocarpin auf den vestibulaeren nystagmus. *Pflügers Archiv* 295:201-204.

Kleitman, N (1925). Studies on the physiology of sleep. III. The effect of muscular activity, rest and sleep on the urinary excretion of phosphorus. *American Journal of Physiology* 74:225-237.

Kleitman, N (1927). Studies on the physiology of sleep. V. Some experiments on puppies. *American Journal of Physiology* 84:386-395.

Kleitman, N (1929). Sleep. *Physiological Reviews* 9:624-665.

Kleitman N (1930). The effect of continued stimulation of sleep upon conditioned salivation. *American Journal of Physiology* 94:215-219.

Kleitman, N (1932). New methods for studying motility during sleep. *Proceedings of the Society for Experimental Biology* 29:389-391.

Kleitman, N (1933). Studies on the physiology of sleep. VIII. Diurnal variation in performance. *American Journal of Physiology* 104:449-456.

Kleitman, N (1939). *Sleep and wakefulness. As alternating phases in the cycle of existence.* Chicago: The University Of Chicago Press.

Kleitman, N (1940). The modifiability of the diurnal pigmentary rhythm in isopods. *Biological Bulletin* 78:403-406.

Kleitman, N (1943). A scientific solution of the multiple shift problem. *Mining Congress Journal* 1943:15-16.

Kleitman, N (1944). Basal temperature grafts and ovulation. *Journal of American Medical Association* (JAMA) 125:82.

Kleitman, N (1945). The effect of motion pictures on body temperature. *Science* 101:507-508.

Kleitman, N (1949a). Mental hygiene of sleep in children. *Nervous Child* 8:63-66.

Kleitman, N (1949b). Biological rhythms and cycles. *Physiological Reviews* 29:1-30.

Kleitman, N (1949c). The sleep-wakefulness cycle in submarine personnel. In: H*uman factors in undersea warfare.* Washington, Nature Research Council, pp 329-341.

Kleitman, N (1950). The sleep-wakefulness cycle. In: *Problem of consciousness*, vol. 1 New-York, Macy, J. Jr. Foundation Conferences. pp 15-60.

Kleitman, N (1952). Modifiability of the diurnal temperature and heart rate curves. *Federation Proceedings* 11:83.

Kleitman, N (1955). The role of the cerebral cortex in the development and maintenance of consciousness. In: Macy, J. Jr *ed., Problem of consciousness: Transactions of the fifth conference. New-York,* Macy, J. Jr. Foundation Conferences, pp 111-132.

Kleitman, N (1957). Sleep, wakefulness, consciousness. *Psychological Bulletin* 54:354-359.

Kleitman, N (1961). The nature of dreaming. In: *The Nature of Sleep.* Wolstenhome G E W, O'Connor M eds. Boston, Ciba Foundation, pp 349-374.

Kleitman, N (1963). *Sleep and Wakefulness.* Chicago-London: The University of Chicago Press.

Kleitman, N (1967a). Phylogenetic, ontogenetic and environmental determinants in the evolution of sleep-wakefulness cycles. In: *Sleep and altered states of consciousness.* Kety S S, Evarts EV, Williams HL, eds. New-York: Williams and Wilkins Company: pp 30-38.

Kleitman, N (1967b). The basic rest-activity cycle and physiological correlates of dreaming. In: Clemente CD ed., *Physiological correlates of dreaming. Experimental Neurology* 19, Suppl. 4:2-4.

Kleitman, N (1972). Introductory remarks. In: *First International Congress of Association for psychophysiological Study of Sleep* Chase M H, ed. Bruges: Brain Research Institute UCLA, p 15

Kleitman, N (1982). Basic rest-activity cycle-22 years later. *Sleep* 5:311-317.

Kleitman, N (1993). Basic rest-activity cycle. In: *Encyclopedia of sleep and dreaming* Carskadon M A ed. New-York: Macmillan, pp 65-66.

Kleitman, N, Blier, ZA (1928). Color and form discrimination in the periphery of the retina. *American Journal of Physiology* 85:178-190.

Kleitman, N, Camille, N (1932). Studies on the physiology of sleep: VI. Behavior of decorticated dogs. *American Journal of Physiology* 100:474-480.

Kleitman, N, Cooperman, NR, Mullin, FJ (1933). Studies on the physiology of sleep. IX. Motility and body temperature during sleep. *American Journal of Physiology* 105:574-584.

Kleitman, N, Crisler, G (1927). Quantitative study of salivary conditioned reflex. *American Journal of Physiology* 79:571-614.

Kleitman, N, Doktorsky, A (1933). Studies on the physiology of sleep. VII. The effect of the position of the body and of sleep on rectal temperature in man. *American Journal of Physiology* 104:340-343.

Kleitman, N, Engelmann, T (1947). Diurnal cycle in activity and body temperature. *Federation Proceedings* 6:143.

Kleitman, N, Engelmann, T (1951). Sleep pattern of infants. *Federation Proceedings* 10:73-74.

Kleitman, N, Engelmann, TG (1953). Sleep characteristics of infants. *Journal of Applied Physiology* 6:269-282.

Kleitman, N, Jackson, DL (1950). Body temperature and performance under different routines. *Journal of Applied Physiology* 3:309-328.

Kleitman, N, Kleijn de, A P H A (1924). The influence of asphyxia on vestibular nystagmus and an attempt to localize the seat of this influence in the reflex arc. *American Journal of Physiology* 69: 160-168.

Kleitman, N, Kleitman, E (1953). Effect of non-twenty-four-hour routines of living on oral temperature and heart rate. *Journal of Applied Physiology* 6:283-291.

Kleitman, N, Kleitman, H (1953). The sleep-wakefulness pattern in the artic. *The Scientific Monthly* 76:349-356.

Kleitman, N, Magnus, R (1924a). Beitrage zur pharmakologie der Koerperstellung und der Labyrinthreflexe. X Mitteilung. Asphyxie. *Pflügers Archiv* 205:142-147.

Kleitman, N, Magnus, R (1924b). Beitrage zur pharmakologie der Koerperstellung und der Labyrinthreflexe. XI Mitteilung. Zur Wirkung des Insulins auf das Zentralnervensystem. *Pflügers Archiv* 205:148-154.

Kleitman, N, Piéron, H (1924a). Loi de variation de la durée de la première phase dans l'établissement de la sensation pour les excitations lumineuses croissantes des cônes et des batonnets. *Comptes Rendus des Séances de la Société de Biologie* 111:456-459.

Kleitman, N, Piéron, H (1924b). Des différences spécifiques entre les cônes et les batonnets dans l'établissement de la sensation lumineuse. *Comptes Rendus des Séances de la Société de Biologie* 111:524-527.

Kleitman, N, Piéron, H (1925). De l'existence de constantes spécifiques différentes pour les radiations chromatiques fondamentales dans l'établissement de la sensation lumineuse par excitation exclusive des cônes rétiniens. *Comptes Rendus des Séances de la Société de Biologie* 112:26-29.

Kleitman, N, Piéron, H (1928). Contribution à l'étude des facteurs régissant le taux de sommation des impressions lumineuses de surface inégales. *L'Année Psychologique* 29:57-91.

Kleitman, N, Ramsaroop, A (1946). Body temperature and cutaneous sensitivity to tingling and pain. *Federation Proceedings* 5:56.

Kleitman, N, Ramsaroop, A (1948). Periodicity in body temperature and heart rate. *Endocrinology* 43:1-20.

Kleitman, N, Ramsaroop, A, Engelmann, T (1948). Variations in skin temperatures of the feet and hands and the onset of sleep. *Federation Proceedings* 7:66.

Kleitman, N, Schreider, JE (1951). Diurnal variation in oculomotor performance. *L'Année Psychologique* 50:201-215.

Kleitman, N, Titelbaum, S, Feiveson, P (1935). Diurnal variation in reaction time and its relation to body temperature. *American Journal of Physiology* 113:82.

Kleitman, N, Titelbaum, S, Feiveson, P (1938). The effect of body temperature on reaction time. *American Journal of Physiology* 121:495-501.

Kleitman, N, Titelbaum, S, Hoffmann, H (1937). The establishment of diurnal temperature cycle. *American Journal of Physiology* 119:48-54.

Kovalzon, VM (2012). Manaseina, Pavlov and the russian school. *European Sleep Research Society 1972-2012*, 40th Anniversary of the ESRS. Bassetti, CL et al. (Eds). Wecom Gesellschaft Kommünikation mbh & Co. Hildesheim:59-60.

Kripke, DF (1978). Wrist actography measures of sleep and rhythms. *Electroencephalography and Clinical Neurophysiology* 44:674-676.

Kubota, K (1989). Kuniomi Ishimori and the first discovery of sleep-inducing substances in the brain. *Neuroscience Research* 6:497-518.

Ladd, GT (1892). Contribution to the psychology of visual dreams. *Mind* 1:299-304.

Lahmeyer, HW (1988) Sleep in craniopagus twins. *Sleep* 11: 301-306.

Lee, MA, Kleitman, N (1923). Studies on the physiology of sleep. II. Attempts to demonstrate functional changes in the nervous system during experimental insomnia. *American Journal of Physiology* 67:141-152.

Legendre, R (1911). La physiologie du sommeil. *La Revue Scientifique* 24:742-751.

Legendre, R, Piéron, H (1907a). Les rapports entre les conditions physiologiques et les modifications histologiques des cellules cérébrales dans l'insomnie expérimentale. *Comptes Rendus des Séances de la Société de Biologie* 62:312-314.

Legendre, R, Piéron, H (1907b). Retour à l'état normal des cellules nerveuses après les modifications provoquées par l'insomnie expérimentale. *Comptes Rendus des Séances de la Société de Biologie* 62:1007-1008.

Legendre, R, Piéron, H (1908). Distribution des altérations cellulaires du système nerveux dans l'insomnie expérimentale. *Comptes Rendus des Séances de la Société de Biologie* 64:1102-1104.

Legendre, R, Piéron, H (1910a). Réfutation expérimentale des théories dites "osmotiques" du sommeil. *Comptes Rendus des Séances de la Société de Biologie* 68:962-964.

Legendre, R, Piéron, H (1910b). La théorie de l'autonarcose carbonique comme cause du sommeil et les données expérimentales. *Comptes Rendus des Séances de la Société de Biologie* 68:1014-1015.

Legendre, R, Piéron, H (1910c). Le problème des facteurs du sommeil. Résultats d'injections vasculaires et intra-cérébrales de liquides insomniques. *Comptes Rendus des Séances de la Société de Biologie* 68:1077-1079.

Legendre, R, Piéron, H (1910d). Des résultats histophysiologiques de l'injection intra-occipito-atlantoïdienne de liquides insomniques. *Comptes Rendus des Séances de la Société de Biologie* 68:1108-1109.

Legendre, R, Piéron, H (1911a). Du développement, au cours de l'insomnie expérimentale, de propriétés hypnotoxiques des humeurs en relation avec le besoin croissant de sommeil. *Comptes Rendus des Séances de la Société de Biologie* 70:190-192.

Legendre, R, Piéron, H (1911b). Contribution expérimentale à la physiologie du sommeil. *Comptes Rendus des Séances de l'Académie des Sciences* 152:456-458.

Legendre, R, Piéron, H (1911c). Effets de la fatigue musculaire sur les cellules du système nerveux central. *Journal de Physiologie Pathologique Générale* 13:519-526.

Legendre, R, Piéron, H (1912a). De la propriété hypnotoxique des humeurs développée au cours d'une veille prolongée. *Comptes Rendus des Séances de la Société de Biologie* 72:210-212.

Legendre, R, Piéron, H (1912b). Destruction par oxydation de la propriété hypnotoxique des humeurs, développée au cours d'une veille prolongée. *Comptes Rendus des Séances de la Société de Biologie* 72:274-275.

Legendre, R, Piéron, H (1912c). Insolubilité dans l'alcool et solubilité dans l'eau de l'"hypnotoxinc" engendrée par une veille prolongée. *Comptes Rendus des Séances de la Société de Biologie* 722:302-304.

Legendre, R, Piéron, H (1913). Recherches sur le besoin de sommeil consécutif à une veille prolongée. *Zeitung für Allgemeine Physiologie* 14:235-262.

Le Grand, H. (1966). Obituary. Henri Piéron (1881-1964). *Vision Research* 6:127-128.

Lenard, HG, Schulte, FJ (1972). Polygraphic sleep study in craniopague twins (where is the sleep transmitter). *Journal of Neurology, Neurosurgery and Psychiatry* 35: 756-762.

Lhermitte, J, Tournay, A (1927). Rapport sur le sommeil normal et pathologique. *Revue Neurologique* I:751-822.

Lindig, P (1922). Ueber Temperatur und Schlaf. *Deutsche Medizine Wochenschrift* 48:765-767 (quoted by Schnedorf and Ivy 1939).

Lindsley, DB, Bowden, JW, Magoun, HW (1949). Effects upon the EEG of acute injury to the brain stem activating system. *Electroencephalography and Clinical Neurophysiology* 1:475-486.

Lindsley, DB, Schreiner, LH, Knowles, WB, Magoun, HW (1950). Behavioral and eeG changes following chronic brain stem lesions in the cat. *Electroencephalography and Clinical Neurophysiology* 2:483-498.

Littman, R (1971). Henri Piéron and french psychology; a comment on Professor Fraisse's note. *Journal of the History of the Behavioral Sciences* 7:261-268.

Loomis, AL, Harvey, EN, Hobart, GAI (1937). Cerebral states during sleep, as studied by human brain potentials. *Journal of Experimental Psychology* 21:127-144.

Lufkin, B (1968). Letter to the editor. *Psychophysiology* 5:449-450.

Luppi, PH (2012). Michel Jouvet and the Lyon school. *European Sleep Research Society 1972-2012*, 40th Anniversary of the ESRS. Bassetti, CL Knobl B, Schulz H (Eds). Wecom Gesellschaft Kommünikation mbh & Co. Hildesheim: 65-66.

Lust, F (1921). Ueber die Beeinflussung der postenzephalitischen Schlafstoerungen durch temperatursteigede Mittel. *Deutsche Medizine Wochenschrift* 47:1545-1547 (quoted by Schnedorf and Ivy 1939).

Magoun, HW (1948). Coma following midbrain lesions in the monkey. Anatomical records100: 752.

Mahmoudzadeh, M, Dehaene-Lambertz G, Fournier M, Kongolo G, Goudjil S, Dubois J, Grebe R, Wallois F (2013). Syllabic discrimination in premature human infants prior to complete formation of cortical layers. *Proceedings of National Academy of Sciences In press.*

Maire, FW, Patton, HD (1954). Hyperactivity and pulmonary edema from rostral hypothalamic lesions in rats. American Journal of Physiolology 178:315-320.

Manaceine de, M (1894). Quelques observations expérimentales sur l'influence de l'insomnie absolue. *Archives Italiennes de Biologie* 21:322-325.

Manceau, A, Jorda, M (1948) Les centres mésodiencéphaliques du sommeil. *La Semaine des Hôpitaux* 24:3193-3202.

Maurel, E (1884). Expériences sur les variations nycthémérales de la température normale. *Comptes Rendus des Séances de la Société de Biologie:* 588.

Mauthner, L (1890). Zur Pathologie und Physiologie des Schlafes. *Wiener Klinische Wochenschrift* 3:445-446.

McGinty, DJ (1969). Somnolence, recovery following ventromedial diencephalic lesion in the rat. *Electroencephalography and clinical Neurophysiology* 26: 70-79.

McGinty, DJ, Sterman, M (1968). Sleep suppression after basal forebrain lesions in the cat. *Science* 160:1253-1255.

Moruzzi, G. (1963). Active processes in the brain during sleep. *The Harvey Lectures*. 56: 233-297

Moruzzi, G (1964). The historical development of the deafferentation hypothesis of sleep. *Proceeedings of American Philosophic Society* 108:19-28.

Moruzzi, G (1972). The sleep-waking cycle. *Ergibnisse der Physiologie,* Berlin: Springer-Verlag. pp 1-165

Moruzzi, G, Magoun, HW (1949). Brain stem reticular formation and activation of the EEG. *Electroencephalography and Clinical Neurophysiolology* 1:455-473.

Mullin, FJ, Kleitman, N (1938). Variations in threshold of auditory stimuli necessary to awaken the sleeper. *American Journal of Physiology* 123:477-481.

Mullin, FJ, Kleitman, N, Cooperman, NR (1933). Studies on the physiology of sleep. X. The effect of alcohol and caffeine on motility and body temperature during sleep. *American Journal of Physiology* 106:478-487.

Mullin, FJ, Kleitman, N, Cooperman, NR (1937). Study on the physiology of sleep. Changes in irratibility to auditory stimuli during sleep. *Journal of Experimental Psychology* 21:88-96.

Nauta, WJH (1946). Hypothalamic regulation of sleep in rats: an experimental study. *Journal of Neurophysiology* 9: 285-316.

Nielsen, T (2000). cognition in REM and NREM sleep: A review and possible reconciliation of two models of sleep mentation. *Behavioral Brain Sciences* 23:851-866.

Noizet, G (1965). Henri Piéron et la promotion de la psychologie. *Cahiers de Psychologie* 8: 1-9.

Pappenheimer, JR, Koski, G, Fencl, V, Karnosky, MI, Krueger, JM (1975) Extraction of sleep-promoting factor S from cerebrospinal fluid and from brains of sleep-deprived animals. *Journal of Neurophysiology* 38:1299-1311.

Patrick, GTW, Gilbert, JA (1896). On the effects of loss of sleep. *Psychological Review* 3:469-483.

Pavlov, I (1954). Oeuvres choisies. Moscou: Editions Langues Etrangères.

Piaget, J (1966). Henri Piéron:1881-1964. *American Journal of Psychology* 69:147-150.

Piéron, H (1901). Sur l'interprétation des faits de rapidité anormale dans le processus d'évocation des images (On the interpretation of facts of abnormal speed in the process of image evocation). In Janet P (Ed) *IVe Congrès International de Psychologie*, Paris, Félix Alcan:439-448). (Quoted by Le Grand Y).

Piéron, H (1904a). De l'immobilité protectrice chez les animaux. *Revue Scientifique* 1:523-527.

Piéron, H (1904b). Du rôle du sens musculaire dans l'orientation de certaines espèces de fourmis. *Bulletin* de l'*Institut Général Psychologique* 168-185.

Piéron, H (1906). La réaction aux marées par anticipation réflexe. *Comptes Rendus des Séances de la Société de Biologie* 61:658-660.

Piéron, H (1907a). La question des rythmes spontanés et des phénomènes d'anticipation en biologie. *Comptes Rendus des Séances de la Société de Biologie* 62:86-88.

Piéron, H (1907b). L'étude expérimentale des facteurs de sommeil normal. La méthode. *Comptes Rendus des Séances de la Société de Biologie* 62:307-309.

Piéron, H (1907c). Comment se pose expérimentalement le problème des facteurs de sommeil. *Comptes Rendus des Séances de la Société de Biologie* 62:342-344.

Piéron, H (1907d) L'état actuel du problème des facteurs du sommeil périodique. I. Insuffisance des voies d'introduction péritlnéale, rachidienne et ventriculaire. *Comptes Rendus des Séances de la Société de Biologie* 62:400-402.

Piéron, H (1907e). Le problème des facteurs de sommeil périodique. *Comptes Rendus des Séances de la Société de Biologie* 62:1005-1007.

Piéron, H (1907f). Des phénomènes d'adaptation biologique par anticipation rythmique. *Comptes Rendus des Séances de la Société de Biologie* 64:338-341.

Piéron, H (1907g). L'adaptation à la recherche du nid chez les fourmis. *Comptes Rendus des Séances de la Société de Biologie* 42:216.

Piéron, H (1908a). La polygenèse des états de sommeil. *Comptes Rendus des Travaux de l'Association Française pour l'Avancement des Sciences*, Session 36, Reims 252-253 .

Piéron, H (1908b). Contribution à l'étude des phénomènes sensoriels et du comportement des vertébrés inférieurs. *Bulletin* de l'*Institut Général Psychologique* 44:322-327.

Piéron, H (1908c). L'évolution du psychisme. *La Revue du Mois* 27:291-310.

Piéron, H (1908d). Contribution à l'étude de l'immobilité protectrice. *Comptes Rendus des Séances de la Société de Biologie* 44:211-213.

Piéron, H (1908e). De l'influence de l'oxygène dissous sur le comportement des invertébrés marins. *Comptes Rendus des Séances de la Société de Biologie* 44:886-888.

Piéron, H (1908f). De l'influence réciproque des phénomènes respiratoires et du comportement chez certaines actinies. *Comptes Rendus de l'Académie des Sciences* 147:1407-1410.

Piéron, H (1908g). La localisation du sens de discrimination alimentaire chez les Limnées. *Comptes Rendus de l'Académie des Sciences* 147:270-280.

Piéron, H (1908h). Le sens chimique des Limnées. *Comptes Rendus des Travaux du Congrès de l' l'Association Française pour l'Avancement des Sciences*, Clermont-Ferrand 82-83.

Piéron, H (1908i). Sur la réflexométrie clinique. Le réflexe patellaire. *Bulletin de la Société de Clinique de Médecine Mentale* 1:20-22.

Piéron, H (1909a). Contribution à la biologie de la Patelle et de la Calyptrée. Le sens du retour et la mémoire topographique. *Archives de Zoologie Expérimentale* 5:18-29.

Piéron, H (1909b). Sens de l'orientation et mémoire topographique de la Patelle. *Comptes Rendus de l'Académie des Sciences* 168:279-280.

Piéron, H (1910a). *L'évolution de la mémoire*. Paris: Flammarion.

Piéron, H (1910b). Contribution à la Biologie de la Patelle et de la Calyptrée. *Bulletin Scientifique de la France et de Belgique* 18:183-202.

Piéron, H (1910c). L'analyse du réflexe rotulien. *Revue Neurologique* 23:597-599.

Piéron, H (1910d). La notion d'exagération du réflexe patellaire et la réflexométrie. *Revue Neurologique* 20:398-402.

Piéron, H (1910e). Le rythme des attitudes mimiques chez un Phasmide (Orthoptère), Le Dixippus Morosus. *Bulletin du Muséum d'Histoire Naturelle* 4:193-196.

Piéron, H (1912). *Le problème physiologique du sommeil.* Doctoral thesis. Paris, Masson.

Piéron, H (1913a). *Le problème physiologique du sommeil.* Paris: Masson.

Piéron, H (1913b). Le sommeil. *Biologia* 38:289-298.

Piéron, H (1914). Recherche sur les lois de variation des temps de latence sensorielle en fonction des intensités excitatrices. *L'Année Psychologique* 22:17-96.

Piéron, H (1927). Discussion du rapport (de Jean Lhermitte and Auguste Tournay). *Revue Neurologique* I:830-832.

Piéron, H (1952). Le phénomène de l'audition atonale dans le sommeil léger. *L'Année Psychologique* 52:393-395.

Piéron, H (1958). *De l'actinie à l'Homme.* Paris: Presses Universitaires de France.

Piéron, H (1965). Discours d'Henri Piéron pour le 75ème anniversaire du laboratoire de Psychologie de la Sorbonne. *L'Année Psychologique* 65:6-15.

Poirier, J, Clarac, F, Barbara, JG, Broussolle, E (2012). Figures and institutions of the neurological sciences in Paris from 1800 to 1950. Part IV: Psychiatry and psychology. *Revue Neurologique* 168: 389-402

Pugnat, CA (1901). Recherches sur les modifications histologiques des cellules nerveuses dans la fatigue. *Journal de Physiologie et de Pathologie Générale* 3:183-187.

Raehlmann, E, Witkowski, L (1877). Ueber atypische Augenbewegungen. *Archiv für Anatomie und Physiologie* S:454-471.

Raehlmann, E, Witkowski, L (1878). Ueber das Verhalten der pupilen während des Schlafen. Nebst Bemerkungen zur Innervation der iris. *Archiv für Anatomie und Physiologie* S: 109-121.

Ranson, SW (1939). Somnolence caused by hypothalamic lesion in the monkey. *Archives of Neurology and Psychiatry of Chicago* 41:1-23.

Reed, CI, Kleitman, N (1926). Studies of the physiology of sleep. IV. The effect of sleep on respiration. *American Journal of Physiology* 75:600-608.

Reuchlin, M (1965). Henri Piéron. *Journal de Psychologie Normale et Pathologique* 62:139-144.

Richter, C (1926). The significance of changes in the electrical resistance of the body during sleep. *Proceedings of National Academy of Sciences* 12: 214-222.

Roffwarg, HP, Dement, WC, Muzio, JN, Fisher, C (1962). Dreaming imagery: relationship to rapid eye movements of sleep. *Archives General of Psychiatry* 7:235-258

Schnedorf, JG, Ivy, AC (1939). An examination of the hypnotoxin theory of sleep. *American Journal of Physiology* 125:491-505.

Schulz, H, Salzarulo, P (2012). Forerunners of REM sleep. *Sleep Medicine Reviews* 16:95-108.

Siegel, JM (2001). A tribute to Nathaniel Kleitman. *Archives Italiennes de Biologie* 139:3-10.

Stefanescu-Goanga, F (1939). Profesorul H. Piéron. *Revista de Psihologie Teoretica si Aplicata* 2:1-4.

Stefanowska, M (1900). Etude histologique du cerveau dans le sommeil provoqué par la fatigue. Journal Belge de Neurologie 5:181-185 (not available).

Steriade, M, McCarley, RW (1990). *Brainstem control of wakefulness and sleep*. New York , Plenum Press.

Sterman, M, Clemente, CD (1962). Forebrain inhibitory mechanisms: sleep patterns induced by basal forebrain stimulation in the behaving cat. *Experimental Neurology* 6:103-117.

Takeuchi, T, Miyasita, A, Inugami, M, Yamamoto, Y (2001). Intrinsic dreams are not produced without REM sleep mechanims : evidence through elicitation of sleep onset periods. *Journal of Sleep Research* 10:43-52.

Takeuchi, T, Ogilvie, RD, Ferrelli, AV, Murphy, T, Yamamoto, Y, Inugami, M (1999). Dreams are not produced without REM sleep mechanisms. *Sleep Research Online* 2 (suppl 1):279.

Toulouse, E, Piéron, H (1906a). Du cycle nycthéméral de la température dans les cas d'activité nocturne et de sommeil diurne. *Comptes Rendus des Séances de la Société de Biologie* 61:473-475.

Toulouse, E, Piéron, H (1906b). Le cycle thermique nycthéméral chez les veilleuses dans leur service de nuit. *Comptes Rendus des Séances de la Société de Biologie* 61:520-522.

Toulouse, E, Piéron, H (1906c). Le passage du cycle nycthéméral normal de la température au cycle inversé. *Comptes Rendus des Séances de la Société de Biologie* 61:558-560.

Toulouse, E, Piéron, H (1907a). La régulation du cycle nycthéméral de la température et son inversion chez les personnes qui veillent. *Comptes Rendus de l'Académie des Sciences* 144:47-49.

Toulouse, E, Piéron, H (1907b). Le mécanisme de l'inversion chez l'Homme. Du rythme nycthéméral de la température. *Journal de Physiologie et de Pathologie Générale* 425-440.

Toulouse, E, Piéron, H (1912). Contribution à l'étude du réflexe rotulien: Réflexes et sommeil- réflexes et bromuration. *Revue de Psychiatrie* 41:271-277.

Toulouse, E, Vaschide, N, Piéron, H (1904). *Technique de Psychologie Expérimentale. Examen des sujets*. Paris, Doin.

Uchizono, K (1984). Studies on sleep substances. *Nihon Rinsho* 42:989-1006.

Vaschide, N (1899). Recherches expérimentales sur les rêves. De la continuité des rêves pendant le sommeil. *Comptes Rendus de l'Académie des Sciences* 129:183-186.

Vaschide, N (1901). Contribution à la séméiologie du rêve. *La Gazette des Hôpitaux* 72-59:569-571.

Vaschide, N (1911). *Le sommeil et les rêves*. Paris, Flammarion.

Vaschide, N, Meunier, P (1901). Projection du rêve dans l'état de veille. *Revue de Psychiatrie* 4:38-49 (not ordered).

Vaschide N, Piéron H (1901a). Prophetic dreams in Greak and Roman antiquity. *The Monist* 161-194.

Vaschide N, Piéron H (1901b). Contribution à la séméiologie du rêve. *La Gazette des Hôpitaux* 74:569-571.

Vaschide N, Piéron H (1902a). *La Psychologie du rêve, au point de vue médical*. Paris, Baillière and Sons.

Vaschide N, Piéron H (1902b). Recherches expérimentales sur la vie mentale d'un xiphophage. *Comptes Rendus de l'Académie des Sciences* 134: 676-678.

Vaschide N, Piéron H (1902c). L'état mental d'un xiphophage. *Revue Scientifique* 555-561.

Vaschide N, Piéron H (1902d). L'état mental d'un xiphophage. *Revue Scientifique* 583-589.

Vaschide N, Vurpas C (1903). Recherches expérimentales sur la psychophysiologie du sommeil. *Comptes Rendus de l'Académie des Sciences* 136:779-782.

Watson J (1972). *Le Behaviorisme*. Paris: Les classiques de la Psychologie.

Webb WB (1978). The sleep of conjoined twins. *Sleep* 1:205-211.

Wikler A (1952). Pharmacological dissociation of behavior and EEG "sleep patterns" in dogs: morphine, N-allylmorphine and atropine. *Proceedings of the Society for Experimental Biology and Medicine* 79:261-265.

Williams HL, Tepas DI, Morlock JHC (1962). Evoked responses to clicks and electroencephalographic stages of sleep in man. *Science* 138:685-686.

Index

#

A

B

C

D

E

F

K

L

M

N

T

U

V

W

Y